The Diversity of the Fungal World

Edited by Jair Putzke

Published in London, United Kingdom

The Diversity of the Fungal World
http://dx.doi.org/10.5772/intechopen.1001506
Edited by Jair Putzke

Contributors
Adolfo Posada, Ali Ebadi, Ana Flávia Zorzi, Ana Luiza Klotz-Neves, Azucena González-Coloma, Caio Henrique Lopes, Charles Xiaoxiang Zhu, Cheewanun Dachoupakan Sirisomboon, Dagoberto Castro, Daniel Rafael Vuelta Lorenzo, Evelise Leis Carvalho, Fernando Augusto Bertazzo-Silva, Flavia Helena Aires Sousa, Gerardo Montero Limonta, Gonfa Kewessa, Jair Putzke, Jorge Renato Pinheiro Velloso, Jorge Rojas López-Menchero, Laura Amália Miranda Costa, Marcos André Pinheiro Velloso, María Fé Andrés-Yeves, Miriela Rizo Mustelier, Mostafa Ebadi, Pablo Martín-Pinto, Panan Rerngsamran, Panmanas Sirisomboon, Rodrigo Patiño, Siannah María Más Diego, Sneha Sharma, Tatek Dejene, Vanielle Galiano, Vicente González-García, Wubalem Tadesse, Xiujuan Yan

First published in London, United Kingdom, 2025 by IntechOpen
IntechOpen is the global imprint of INTECHOPEN LIMITED, registered in England and Wales, registration number: 11086078, 167-169 Great Portland Street, London, W1W 5PF, United Kingdom

For EU product safety concerns: IN TECH d.o.o., Prolaz Marije Krucifikse Kozulić 3, 51000 Rijeka, Croatia, info@intechopen.com or visit our website at intechopen.com.

British Library Cataloguing-in-Publication Data
A catalogue record for this book is available from the British Library

The Diversity of the Fungal World
Edited by Jair Putzke
p. cm.
Print ISBN 978-0-85466-434-4
Online ISBN 978-0-85466-433-7
eBook (PDF) ISBN 978-0-85466-435-1

Meet the editor

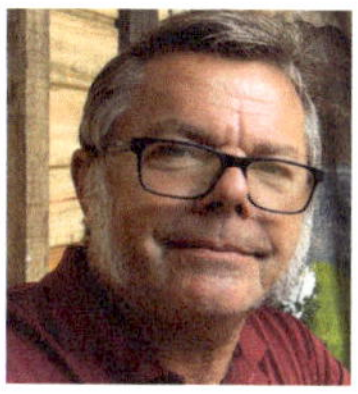

Jair Putzke has a degree in Biological Sciences from the Universidade de Santa Cruz do Sul – Brazil (1990), a master's degree in Cryptogams from the Universidade Federal de Pernambuco – Brazil (1994), and a Ph.D. in Botany from the Federal University of Rio Grande do Sul – Brazil (2003). He is currently a professor at the Universidade Federal do Pampa (UNIPAMPA) - São Gabriel campus in Southern Brazil. He has experience in Botany with an emphasis on Mycology, working mainly on the following topics: fungi taxonomy, ecology and phytogeography, myxomycetes taxonomy and ecology, Antarctic cryptogams and environmental education. Now associated with the Postgraduate Course in Biological Sciences at UNIPAMPA, he is doing research in Southern Brazil, in the Amazon biome, Andes and Antarctica. He has about 140 scientific articles, 25 books and 18 book chapters published.

Contents

Preface

Fungi organisms are increasingly recognized as essential to the functioning of our ecosystems and as practical uses for our benefit. They increasingly fascinate scientists, from their function as nutrient cyclers to their relationships with other organisms. How can one get to know the world of fungi if one does not yet know their diversity? Basic studies still need to be accomplished in many countries worldwide, and new revelations in the molecular field show that we are very far from completing this issue.

Some continents still do not have their fungi known, not even in the most apparent groups, such as those that form macroscopic reproductive structures; imagine the numbers in the microscopic ones! And what is the knowledge regarding its interactions with other organisms? No book can cover everything already known about fungi, but they are important for directing scientific progress, even when revising what is already known, and for attracting and inspiring both the general public and the scientific community while maintaining proper balance.

It is urgent to explore fungal diversity before it disappears due to the anthropogenic attacks of all kinds that it has been suffering, extinguishing species before they are even known. And the kingdom of fungi has the greatest yet unknown diversity among the different groups. Searching for unknown species requires a huge investment in training new taxonomists in each country. However, fewer and fewer mycologists and taxonomists are being prepared each year. The emphasis has been on other areas, aiming for an immediate use of the species, not always to preserve them. Massive studies focus on the usual or most frequent species, and knowledge about those recently described or already named is incipient.

Previously, giant forests, savannas, and open fields across the planet disappeared, but now they disappear more quickly due to uncontrolled and large-scale fires all around the planet. The loss of fungal diversity due to the recent fires in Australia, Europe, the Amazon, and North America is invaluable. We often despair over the loss of animals or trees in disasters like these, but most people don't realize that microscopic organisms hold the largest and most fragile biodiversity. Protecting these groups of organisms depends on basic studies. The protection of these groups of organisms is dependent on basic studies.

Climate change is bringing all this diversity to an even faster end. Increases in average temperature, severe droughts in specific regions and intense rains in others also affect fungal biodiversity. The impacts are still being discovered, but the effect on a global level is difficult to estimate. Plant diseases are becoming increasingly common and may also be associated with these events. New phytopathogenic fungi control techniques, including those that do not use toxic substances, are needed.

As a result, the opportunity arises to launch a book with the most current information on the diversity and interrelationships of fungi species and fungi associated with other groups of organisms, with the collaboration of scientists from different regions of the planet.

In this regard came the invaluable contributions to this book from all continents. A first review of fungi from Ethiopia is presented, with data on distribution, threats and prospects. Revisions on the knowledge of each country's fungi are essential to encourage other scientists to contribute to the list's survey and enrichment and establish the starting point of new revisionary works. Many African countries still have no checklist on fungi, so a chapter like this is a stimulus to new surveys in this area.

The chapters on endophyte fungi, those associated with the living tissue of plants but without causing any disease, cover taxonomy, isolation and identification methods, in addition to molecular studies and metagenomics works involving the group. The potential for biotechnological application of key species is also discussed, mainly for soil restoration, plant protection and disease control.

Other chapters discuss aspects of phytopathology involving fungi. One of them discusses using near-infrared hyperspectral images to detect anthracnose in mango. This technique is proving to be an efficient alternative for rapidly detecting fruit pathogens, depending on the change in temperature in the infected areas. Another one discussed the mycorrhizal fungi and magnetically treated water to biocontrol nematodes. All recent techniques are fully revised, and we are waiting for more research using other areas and substrates.

With all these contributions, this book aims to help find fungi worldwide, giving the steps on how to study some of their groups and how to control the pathogenic ones using non-toxic techniques. So that the studies of fungi can be stimulated worldwide, attracting new taxonomists and people interested in the practical application of fungi.

The authors wish to thank the director of the Universidade Federal do Pampa (UNIPAMPA), campus São Gabriel, Dr. Luciana Borba Benetti, for the support of the activities that resulted in this book; to the Laboratório de Taxonomia de Fungos – LATAF (UNIPAMPA) staff for their technical support; the Coordenação de Aperfeiçoamento de Pessoal de Nível Superior – Brazil (CAPES – Finance Code 001) for granting a scholarship to some of the authors; the Fundação de Amparo à Pesquisa do Rio Grande do Sul, Southern Brazil (FAPERGS - project no. 21/2551-0001985-9) for the resources granted; and the Conselho Nacional de Pesquisa e Desenvolvimento Científico e Tecnológico (CNPq - project no. 405564/2022-8) for the financial support; and to Universal Funga do Brazil Project, coordinated by Dr. Elisandro Ricardo Drechsler-Santos for the support provided (project no. 403547/2023-7).

Jair Putzke
Universidade Federal do Pampa (UNIPAMPA),
São Gabriel, Brazil

Section 1

Fungal Diversity and Interactions

Chapter 1

Fungal Biodiversity in Ethiopia: Distribution, Threats and Prospects

Gonfa Kewessa, Tatek Dejene, Wubalem Tadesse and Pablo Martín-Pinto

Abstract

Fungi are an integral part of the natural world, playing important roles in ecological processes and having considerable potential for use in diverse industries. Despite the rich fungal diversity in Ethiopia, limited information exists regarding their distribution, threats, and conservation efforts. Even, fungi are not included in the biodiversity database of the country. This chapter provides a synthesis of information gathered from different sources to understand fungal biodiversity, focusing on the distributions, threats to and conservation of fungal species across various land uses and sites in Ethiopia. The fungal biodiversity in the country is extensive, encompassing a wide range of fungal species. However, fungi in Ethiopia are threatened by multiple factors, including land use/land cover changes, deforestation, habitat degradation, the expansion of invasive plant species, and climate change. This leads to effective conservation and management of biodiversity to ensure their sustainable use, thus enhancing the resilience and productivity of habitats, different ecosystems, and mycological resources. To this end, this chapter will contribute to the existing body of knowledge and help in the formulation of strategies for sustainable management of fungal biodiversity.

Keywords: Ethiopia, biodiversity conservation, rural people, mycological resources, nonwood forest products

1. Introduction

Fungi constitute one of the most diverse groups of organisms on Earth, second only to insects in terms of diversity [1]. Fungi play crucial roles in ecosystems as decomposers, symbionts with animals and plants, and parasites, thus enabling life on Earth [2]. Mushrooms, which are seasonal fungi, occupy diverse niches in forest ecosystems and are vital to all ecosystems [3, 4]. Understanding their ecological distribution is essential for effective conservation and sustainable management strategies.

According to the latest estimates, the total number of fungal species worldwide is believed to be between 2.2 million and 3.8 million [5]. However, only approximately 148,000 species have been formally described and named. This vast discrepancy highlights the immense diversity of fungi and the significant number of species yet to be discovered and classified. The estimates continue to evolve as new species are discovered and as molecular techniques improve our understanding of fungal biodiversity. Several mycologists have attempted to answer the question of "Where are the missing fungi?" by identifying the habitats that are to be studied for the presence of such fungi [6].

Forests are among the most promising habitats for exploring these "missing" fungi. They serve as vital reservoirs of biodiversity, housing a myriad of plant and animal species crucial for ecosystem functioning and human well-being. Among these diverse organisms, fungi stand out as a significant component of forest ecosystems, playing key roles in nutrient cycling, decomposition processes, and symbiotic relationships with other organisms.

Given the global importance of forests for fungal biodiversity, Ethiopia is particularly significant due to its rich and diverse vegetation resources that range from lowland scrubs to tropical rainforests [7]. These diverse forest types provide a unique opportunity to study a wide array of fungal species, each contributing uniquely to the ecological tapestry of the region. Moreover, Ethiopia's forests are under various threats, including deforestation and climate change, making the understanding and conservation of fungal biodiversity even more critical.

To address these concerns, this chapter provides a synthesis of information to understand fungal biodiversity in Ethiopia, focusing on fungal distributions, threats to and conservation of fungal species across various land uses and sites. Information about the distribution and diversity of fungi, threats and prospects will lead to effective management of biodiversity and ensure their sustainable use, thus enhancing the resilience and productivity of Ethiopia's forest ecosystems and mycological resources.

2. Methodology

Our methodology involves collecting and analyzing available literature, research reports, and datasets related to fungal diversity in natural and plantation forests in Ethiopia. We performed a systematic literature review of scientific databases such as PubMed, Scopus, and Web of Science using relevant keywords such as "fungi" and paired search terms such as "fungal threats in Ethiopia" and "fungal distribution in Ethiopia" to identify articles and studies related to the topic of interest, as described in previous studies [8]. A total of 150 articles were downloaded for this study. After a thorough review and evaluation of their relevance and quality, 63 of these articles were selected and utilized as the main sources. These selected articles provided the foundational information and critical insights necessary for synthesizing the content of this chapter. Then, in this chapter, we synthesize existing data and information to provide a comprehensive overview of fungal diversity within various forest systems across Ethiopia. For example, in southern Ethiopia, studies have focused on the diversity and succession of fungal communities in *Pinus patula* [9, 10] and *Eucalyptus grandis* plantations [11, 12], as well as their response to stand development and fire occurrences [10, 13]. Notable studies include investigations into soil fungal communities in various aged plantations and the richness and diversity of macrofungi in natural forests and plantations in Dagaga and Gambo natural and plantation forests [14]. Research in northern Ethiopia has explored macrofungal diversity and the influence of edaphic factors on fungal communities in church forests in Dry Afromontane areas [15], with additional studies utilizing metabarcoding to aid conservation efforts [16]. In northwestern Ethiopia, studies have primarily concentrated on *Termitomyces* species, including morphological and molecular analyses [17] and ethnomycological surveys of edible and medicinal mushrooms in the Menge District [18]. In the central highlands of Ethiopia, research has highlighted the impact of forest type and site conditions on the diversity and biomass of edible macrofungal species [19], with specific studies emphasizing the retention of mature trees in *Pinus radiata* plantations to conserve fungal diversity [20] and documenting new records of *Agaricus* species [21]. These regional studies and the synthesis of previous research provide valuable insights into the current understanding of fungal biodiversity across varied landscapes in Ethiopia.

3. Fungal biodiversity in Ethiopia

Ethiopia has a wide range of ecological, climatic, and geographical conditions, including highlands, lowlands, and various forest types, which are known to support high biodiversity levels [22]. The country's rich plant, animal, and microbial genetic resource diversity, along with its ecosystem variability, requires serious protection, conservation, and management to derive sustainable benefits for present and future generations. Although Ethiopia is home to a diverse range of fungal species [23–25], many of these species remain unidentified or undiscovered.

Our extensive research over the years has meticulously analyzed the fungal diversity and composition in natural forests, particularly fragmented church forests, and plantations in Ethiopia, which are primarily dominated by pines and eucalyptus. The findings from our studies on fruiting bodies highlight the significant ecological richness in natural forests, where we identified up to 188 distinct taxa [15]. Remarkably, 81% of these taxa are saprotrophic fungi that play a crucial role in decomposing organic matter, while 14% are ECM (ectomycorrhizal) fungi [15], which form beneficial symbiotic relationships with tree roots. Another study revealed a total of 61 fungal taxa belonging to the Basidiomycota division [26]. This diversity underscores the ecological complexity and resilience of natural forest ecosystems. Conversely, plantations exhibited a substantially lower number of taxa, with 53 in pine forests and 29 in eucalyptus plantations [12]. Despite this reduced diversity, pine plantations contained 36% edible species, highlighting their potential for sustainable foraging and local food resources. Additionally, by analyzing the soil fungal communities, the results provide profound ecological insights into the fungal diversity within natural forests and plantations dominated by dominant pine and *eucalyptus* species. In fragmented natural forests, we observed 2898 operational taxonomic units (OTUs), with 52% belonging to Ascomycota and 20% to Basidiomycota, the two primary phyla [13]. Similarly, in pine-dominated forest stands, 2262 OTUs were identified [9], while *Eucalyptus* forests hosted 2886 OTUs, with 47% being saprotrophs and 15% being ECM fungi, the predominant guilds [11]. These findings underscore the remarkable diversity present within Ethiopian forest ecosystems. The high number of OTUs and the prevalence of diverse fungal phyla and guilds highlight the ecological complexity and richness of these ecosystems. Furthermore, the dominance of Ascomycota and Basidiomycota underscores their fundamental roles in nutrient cycling and ecosystem functioning. The prevalence of saprotrophs and ECM fungi indicates their crucial functions in organic matter decomposition and nutrient exchange with host plants, contributing to ecosystem stability and resilience.

These findings underscore the importance of conserving natural forests due to their rich fungal diversity while also revealing the ecological value of plantation forests in supporting specific fungal communities. Information on fungal distribution across various forest types and land uses enhances our understanding of fungal biodiversity and ecological dynamics across varied landscapes [3, 25]. This understanding is crucial for the careful consideration of unique and shared species across different forest types, ensuring the sustainable use and conservation of fungal biodiversity in Ethiopia's diverse forest ecosystems.

3.1 Edible fungal species in Ethiopia

After obtaining a general understanding of fungal diversity in Ethiopian forests, we also performed a comprehensive evaluation of wild edible mushroom resources. Our study aimed to address two key objectives: first, to document the fresh weight of edible wild mushrooms harvested from the natural and plantation forests in Ethiopia. Second, to construct predictive models for sporocarp production in these distinct forest systems. We found a total of 64 edible fungal species. Notably, the average annual total fresh weight production in plantations (2097.57 kg ha^{-1}) significantly exceeded that in natural forests (731.18 kg ha^{-1}) [19]. As a result, we developed yield classification models to provide a framework for predicting the annual yields of edible fungi based on Ethiopia's specific climatic, soil, and geographical characteristics [27]. These models represent a foundational tool for guiding future research endeavors in Ethiopian forests, facilitating the optimization of forest management strategies centered around NTFPs, particularly edible wild mushrooms.

Mushrooms in Ethiopia can be found in diverse ecological zones, such as highlands, lowlands, and forested areas. Nevertheless, the diversity of Ethiopian mushrooms has not been thoroughly studied or documented across all ecosystems to date [25]. The highlands of Ethiopia are home to several edible mushrooms, including *Pleurotus ostreatus*, *Termitomyces microcarpus*, and *Ramaria* sp. The hot and dry climate of the Rift Valley provides suitable conditions for growing a variety of mushroom species, such as *Termitomyces* sp. and *Auricularia* sp. Some other appreciated mushroom species include *Boletus* sp., *Lactarius* sp., and *Ganoderma* sp. **Figure 1** illustrates some of the most commonly found mushroom species in Ethiopia [14, 23].

The diversity and distribution of mushrooms are significantly influenced by a range of ecological and environmental variables. These factors include forest type, altitudinal gradients, soil characteristics, vegetation cover, interactions with other organisms, and specific temperature and humidity requirements, among others, as detailed below:

Forest type: Different types of forests, such as tropical rainforests, montane forests, and dry forests, harbor distinct fungal communities due to variations in temperature, humidity, and vegetation composition (**Figure 2**). Fungi exhibit preferences for specific habitat niches within different forest types [28–30], influencing their distribution and abundance. Forest type acts as a broad-scale determinant, delineating the overarching environmental conditions that govern fungal community composition [31, 32].

Altitude: Altitudinal gradients in mountainous regions of Ethiopia create diverse microclimates, impacting fungal diversity. Fungal communities often exhibit altitudinal zonation patterns, with species richness and composition changing with elevation [33]. Altitudinal gradients further contribute to fungal diversity, with each elevational band presenting unique climatic conditions and ecological niches. In the Ethiopian highlands, montane forests exhibit distinct fungal communities at different

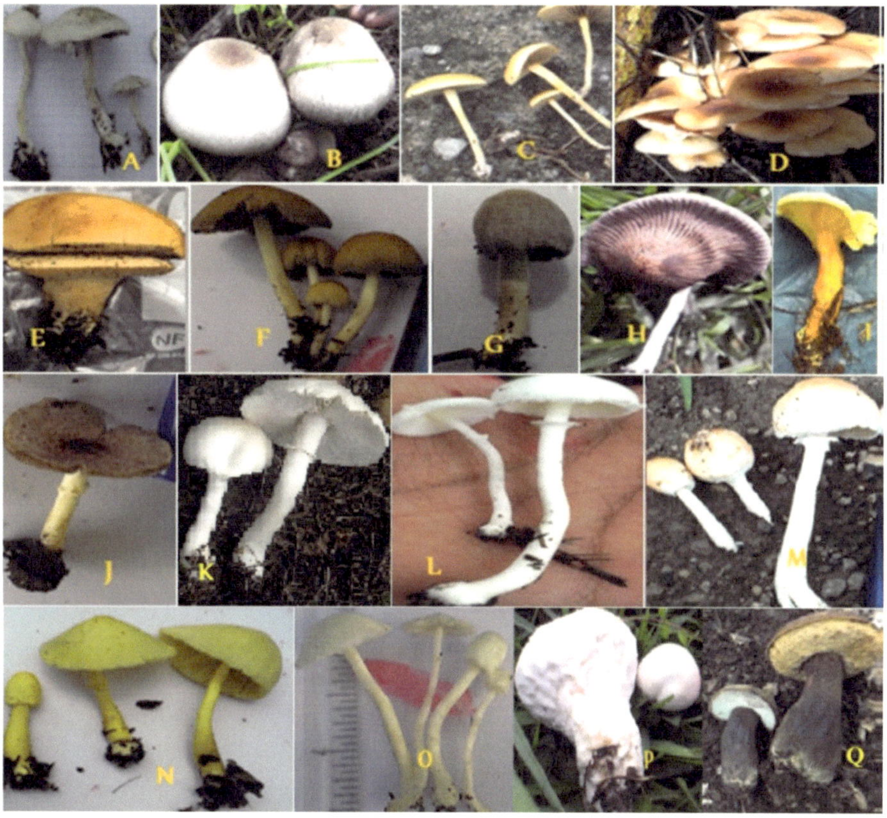

Figure 1.
Photographic representation of 17 selected mushroom species recorded in Ethiopia. The images labeled A to Q correspond to the following species: (A) Agaricus campestroides, (B) Agaricus subedulis, (C) Agrocybe pediades, (D) Armillaria heimii, (E) Calvatia rubroflava, (F) Coprinellus domesticus, (G) Coprinopsis nivea, (H) Coprinus pseudoplicatilis, (I) Hygrophoropsis aurantiaca, (J) Hymenagaricus fuscobrunneus, (K) Leucoagaricus holosericeus, (L) Leucoagaricus leucothites, (M) Leucoagaricus rubrotinctus, (N) Leucocoprinus birnbaumii, (O) Leucocoprinus cepistipes, (P) Lycoperdon perlatum, and (Q) Tylopilus niger.

elevations, ranging from montane forests at higher altitudes to subalpine vegetation at lower elevations.

Soil characteristics: Soil properties, including pH, texture, organic matter content, and nutrient availability, shape fungal communities. Different fungal species exhibit specific adaptations to soil conditions, influencing their distribution across various soil types [16, 27]. Soil characteristics exert profound influences on fungal distribution, reflecting the intricate interactions between fungi and their substrates. The acidic soils prevalent in some Ethiopian forests favor acidophilic fungal species, while nutrient-rich soils support diverse decomposer communities involved in organic matter decomposition and nutrient cycling. One of the primary factors that influences sporocarp production in fungi is the availability of nutrients [34, 35]. Fungi require specific nutrients to grow and reproduce, and the availability of these nutrients can vary depending on the ecological niche of the fungus. For example, some fungi require specific types of organic matter, such as dead wood or leaf litter, to produce sporocarps. Other fungi may require specific types of soil or certain microorganisms to produce sporocarps.

Vegetation cover: The composition and structure of vegetation influence fungal diversity by providing habitat, organic matter, and niche diversity. Fungal

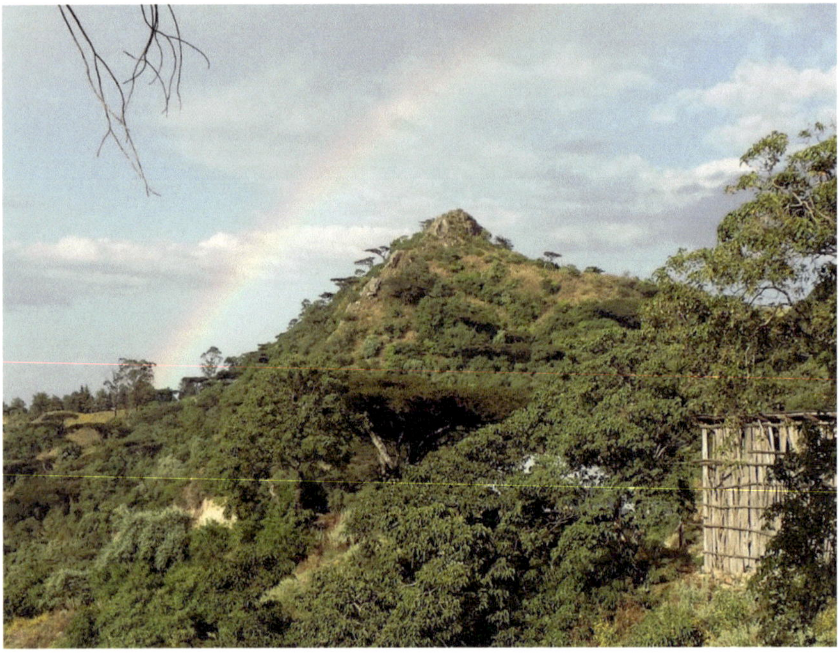

Figure 2.
The wealth of Ethiopian Dry Afromontane forests harboring diverse fungal resources. This figure illustrates the rich fungal biodiversity found within these unique forest ecosystems, highlighting the ecological significance of diverse fungal species.

communities exhibit associations with specific plant species, forming symbiotic relationships or engaging in decomposition processes [30, 36, 37]. Moreover, vegetation cover acts as a key determinant of fungal diversity by providing habitat and resources for fungal growth and reproduction. Forest structure, canopy cover, and plant species composition influence the microclimatic conditions and organic inputs available to fungi, shaping community composition and functional roles.

Relationships with other organisms: Another factor that can influence sporocarp production in fungi is the presence of other organisms in the ecosystem. Fungi often interact with other organisms, such as plants and animals, in complex ways. These interactions can affect the availability of resources for fungi and can also influence the distribution and abundance of fungal species. For example, some fungi may form mutualistic relationships with plants [38–40], where fungi provide nutrients to plants in exchange for carbohydrates. In these cases, the presence of the plant can influence the production of sporocarps by the fungus.

Temperature and humidity: These are also important factors that can influence sporocarp production in fungi [41]. Different fungal species have different temperature and humidity requirements, and these requirements can vary depending on the ecological niche of the fungus. For example, some fungi may require high humidity levels to produce sporocarps, while others may require lower humidity levels [42].

3.2 Ethnomycology of mushrooms in Ethiopia

Globally, ethnomycology has emerged as a significant field of study [43, 44]. This knowledge is a crucial aspect of many communities' identities. Preserving information about the use of wild mushrooms, their linguistic terms, and harvesting methods is crucial to prevent their loss due to modernization and dominant cultures. Documenting this knowledge can promote the revaluation and conservation of wild mushroom species. Revitalizing the knowledge and nomenclature of useful species and encouraging their use could enhance the contribution of wild mushrooms to food security, particularly in Ethiopia, where food security is a national concern.

In many societies, mushrooms serve multiple purposes: they are used as food, medicine, enzymes, and other industrial substances [18, 43, 45]. Additionally, mushrooms hold recreational value and are significant in the myths and beliefs of various cultures [46]. As a nutritious substitute for meat and fish, mushrooms are rich in proteins, vitamins, lipids, carbohydrates, amino acids, and minerals [43, 46, 47]. Locals frequently collect these valuable NTFPs, which help them avoid poverty and sustain their livelihoods [43, 46, 48]. Mushrooms are part of life in their wild form for food, as shown in **Figure 3**.

One of our previous studies [49] aimed to provide baseline information about the ethnomycology of various ethnic groups in Ethiopia. These groups, which are located in the same geographic region, interact with the same natural resources and possess similar knowledge of wild mushrooms. This similarity stems from their cultural exchanges, coexistence, and shared historical events. Many respondents reported that although they do not consume mushrooms themselves, their parents or grandparents do, indicating that mycological knowledge is at risk of being lost among these groups [49]. In contrast, wild mushroom consumption remains an integral part of cultural knowledge regarding seasonal resources in some southern communities. Therefore, further study of traditional food compositions and recipes is necessary to determine the potential nutritional and food security benefits of wild mushrooms for these communities. In areas where mushrooms are commonly used, women primarily gather and collect valuable wild mushrooms, highlighting that gender significantly influences local knowledge and the distribution of wild mushrooms [18, 49]. This has implications for women's contributions to household food security through the use of locally available food resources, such as fungi. Thus, fungi could provide supplementary food, reduce poverty, and offer opportunities for women in unfavorable areas, thereby reducing inequality.

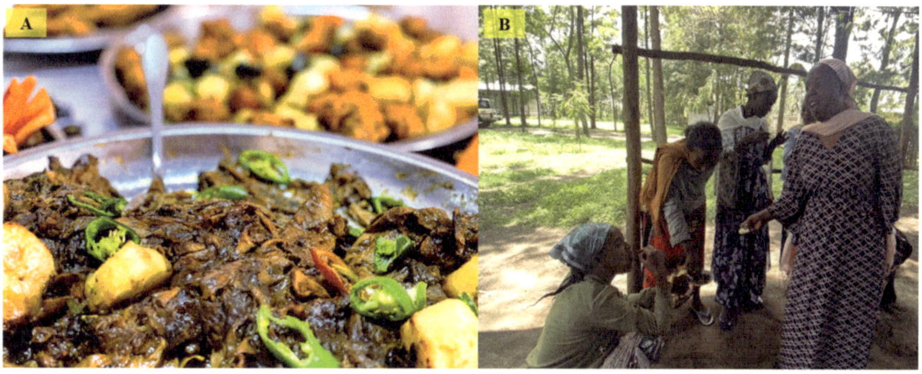

Figure 3.
Image (A) illustrates the culinary versatility of mushrooms, showcasing their preparation and final presentation as a dish. Image (B) shows local community members engaging in communal mushroom foraging, emphasizing the social and economic significance of mushrooms.

4. Threats of fungal species in Ethiopia

Wild mushrooms in Ethiopia face threats without adequate scientific documentation due to factors such as deforestation, forest degradation, land use and land cover changes, climate change, invasive species, and a lack of awareness and conservation efforts. Some of these threats are discussed below.

Deforestation: The loss of forested areas due to agriculture, mining, and other human activities has led to a decline in the natural habitats of mushrooms [50]. This has made it difficult for some species of mushrooms to thrive. Deforestation is a severe threat to mushroom species in Ethiopia because it destroys the natural habitats of many mushrooms [2]. The forests in Ethiopia have diverse ecological niches that support the growth of mushrooms, providing suitable living conditions for many species. When these habitats are destroyed through deforestation, the fungal populations residing in them are also impacted. **Figure 4** illustrates that large-scale tree harvesting for commercial purposes poses a threat to mushroom resources. Deforestation reduces the number of trees and reduces environmental humidity levels, making it challenging for different mushroom species to survive. Additionally, deforestation often leads to soil erosion and nutrient depletion, making the remaining soil inhospitable to fungi and other organisms. Reduced forest cover often results in more drastic fluctuations in temperatures that drive some mushroom species away from their suitable habitats. Thus, disrupted ecosystems and a lack of fungal interactions due to deforestation can also contribute to further disruption of forest biodiversity. Thus, deforestation deprives many mushroom species of vital habitat and threatens their continued existence in Ethiopia. Protecting these ecosystems is necessary to conserve their biodiversity and the important roles these mushrooms play in the ecosystem.

Land degradation: Soil erosion and poor land use practices have also contributed to the loss of suitable habitats for mushrooms. Land degradation is a significant threat to mushroom species in Ethiopia [51]. The loss of soil fertility, erosion, and changes

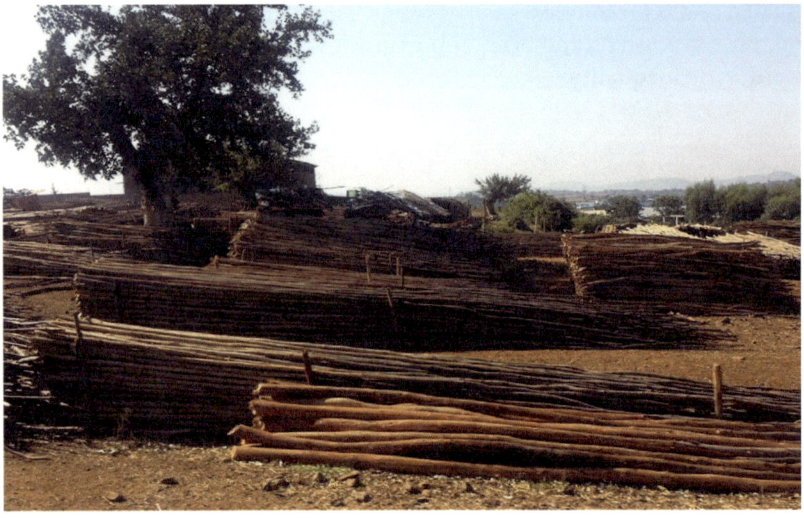

Figure 4.
Large-scale tree harvesting for commercial purposes poses a threat to mushroom resources. The photo illustrates the extensive logging activities that led to habitat loss and degradation, impacting the diversity and abundance of fungal species.

in the physical properties of the soil due to human activities subject mushroom populations to different stress types. These factors modify soil conditions, disrupt natural cycles, and prevent mushroom species from growing healthily. Land degradation is often caused by unsustainable land use practices, such as overgrazing, land conversion, and widespread agricultural practices. For instance, land clearing for agriculture can lead to soil erosion, leaving exposed land that is unsuitable for the growth of edible or medicinal mushrooms. Overgrazing can also cause the soil to be more compact and stripped of nutrients. Soil damage caused by these activities can lead to a change in habitat, making it unsuitable for mushroom species to grow in such an environment [52]. The loss of soil moisture and nutrients, for example, deprives plants of the basic resources needed to survive and produce underground fruiting bodies of mushroom species. Fungal population reduction also leads to reduced decomposition rates of natural organic matter, thereby greatly impacting the habitat's carbon cycle [53]. Moreover, land degradation has a profound impact on the natural habitats of mushroom species, making it difficult for them to survive, reproduce, and support other organisms in the ecosystem. Sustainable land use practices and conservation efforts are necessary to prevent changes in soil conditions from degrading natural habitats that support the growth of mushroom species in Ethiopia.

Overgrazing: Uncontrolled grazing by livestock can damage the soil and reduce the number of edible mushrooms available. Overgrazing is a significant threat to mushroom species in Ethiopia [54]. Overgrazing occurs when too many animals, such as goats, sheep, or cattle, graze on a particular piece of land, causing soil compaction, changes in soil structure, and a reduction in soil moisture. This can have several adverse effects on the growth and development of mushrooms. Overgrazing causes soil compaction, tilting the soil microbiota, and limiting air movement, reducing the soil's ability to hold water, which is necessary to support the growth of mushrooms. This results in a change in soil conditions that affects mushroom habitats and restricts their ability to colonize specific soils. Mushrooms have a symbiotic relationship with plants, where they form connections with roots to exchange nutrients [55]. Overgrazing leads to a reduced availability of plant biomass inside the soil, leading to a decrease in belowground biomass and a decrease in fungal populations [56]. Overgrazing also leads to a reduction in vegetative cover, resulting in increased soil exposure to rain and leading to soil erosion. This exposes the soil to harsh environmental conditions and encourages the spread of invasive plant species that may negatively impact native mushroom populations through competition, habitat destruction potential, and changes in the soil microclimate [57]. Moreover, overgrazing impacts the physical characteristics of the soil and the relationships between mushrooms and host plants and changes the soil microbiota, thus threatening mushroom species diversity and populations and potentially affecting overall ecosystem sustainability in Ethiopia.

Climate change: Changes in temperature and rainfall patterns can have a negative impact on mushroom growth and reproduction. Changes in temperature, rainfall patterns, and water availability can negatively impact the growth and reproduction of mushrooms in several ways. Temperature changes can alter the timing of fruiting body formation, affect fruiting body quality, and make areas unsuitable for some mushroom species. A shifting temperature gradient and moisture can destroy suitable habitats, forcing some species to migrate to cooler climates and restricting the growth of heat-sensitive species [58]. Changes in rainfall patterns can affect the timing of mushroom fruiting, prohibit or promote the growth of some species, and lead to increased competition with other species [59]. Extended dry seasons resulting from erratic rain patterns affect fruiting body development and may lead to a reduction in water availability in the area, which is essential for the growth of many mushroom species. Furthermore, changes in the availability of water in the ecosystem, leading to localized drought or flooding, can affect fruiting body maturity rates. Climate change can also increase the growth of molds, which compete with other beneficial microbial organisms, such as mycorrhizae, for resources and damage fruiting bodies [60]. The changing ecology could promote the invasion of fungal pathogens, leading to a decrease in specialized mushroom species populations and biodiversity. Generally, climate change threatens mushroom species in Ethiopia by altering their habitat, leading to changes in their growth patterns and fruiting habits, and can cause the invasion of harmful fungi, posing significant challenges to ecosystem maintenance and their esthetic importance. Therefore, addressing these threats requires integrated approaches, including public awareness campaigns.

5. Conservation and sustainable forest management measures

5.1 Habitat conservation

Identifying and preserving these diverse habitats is crucial for promoting the conservation of mushrooms and their economic potential in Ethiopia. Therefore, the conservation and sustainable use of forest systems are essential for preserving fungal diversity and promoting ecosystem health in Ethiopian forests. Habitat conservation initiatives, such as protected areas and conservation reserves, provide vital refuges for fungal species, protecting them from habitat destruction and degradation.

To achieve sustainable forest management and prevent *deforestation*, the implementation of several key strategies is crucial. First, it is crucial to promote reforestation by actively planting native tree species to restore degraded areas. Additionally, it is essential to strengthen and enforce laws against illegal logging and land conversion. Supporting the rights of local communities and indigenous peoples, allowing them to manage and protect their forests, is also vital. Encouraging sustainable logging practices and certifying timber products ensures that forest exploitation does not compromise the ecosystem. Utilizing technology, such as satellite imagery, to monitor forest health and illegal activities enhances surveillance and control. Finally, raising public awareness about the importance of forests and sustainable practices is vital to ensuring community support and participation in these efforts.

To prevent *soil degradation*, especially in areas near lakes and water bodies, it is essential to recognize the crucial role that forests play. In these regions, trees and plants act as natural barriers that prevent erosion and maintain water quality. An effective strategy is to use mycorrhizal fungi in plantation plants. These fungi not only help plants adapt to poor soils, enhancing their resistance and growth but also provide a food resource and an intermediate source of income for rural populations. By incorporating these techniques, sustainable forest management can be promoted to protect the natural environment and enhance the economic well-being of local communities while ensuring the preservation of nearby aquatic ecosystems.

The importance of *preventing overgrazing* cannot be overstated, as it can lead to the removal of vegetation, which in turn can cause severe erosion, as previously noted. When vegetation is stripped away, the soil loses its protective cover, making it vulnerable to wind and water erosion. This not only depletes the soil of essential nutrients but also leads to the loss of biodiversity, including vital mycological resources, including appreciated edible mushroom species. The disappearance of fungi that form symbiotic relationships with plants can further degrade the ecosystem, as these fungi are crucial for nutrient cycling and soil health. To combat overgrazing, several measures can be designed and implemented. First, rotational grazing can be introduced, where livestock are moved between pastures to allow vegetation in previously grazed areas to recover. Second, setting up controlled grazing systems with designated grazing periods and rest periods for the land can help maintain vegetation cover. Third, planting cover crops and introducing forage species that are resilient to grazing pressure can help protect the soil. Additionally, implementing buffer zones around sensitive areas, such as water bodies, can prevent livestock from overgrazing these critical zones. Providing alternative feed sources during dry seasons or periods of low vegetation growth can also reduce the pressure on natural pastures. Educating farmers and herders about sustainable grazing practices and the long-term benefits of maintaining healthy ecosystems is essential. Government policies and incentives that support sustainable livestock management can further reinforce these practices. By taking these steps, we can protect vegetation, preserve biodiversity, and maintain the mycological resources necessary for a resilient and productive ecosystem.

To promote sustainable forest management that preserves fungal communities in the face of *climate change*, it is essential to adopt several strategies. Encouraging myco-silviculture, which integrates fungal cultivation into forestry practices, can enhance ecosystem resilience and biodiversity. Adapting forest density to changing climate conditions is crucial; reducing tree density can decrease stress on individual trees,

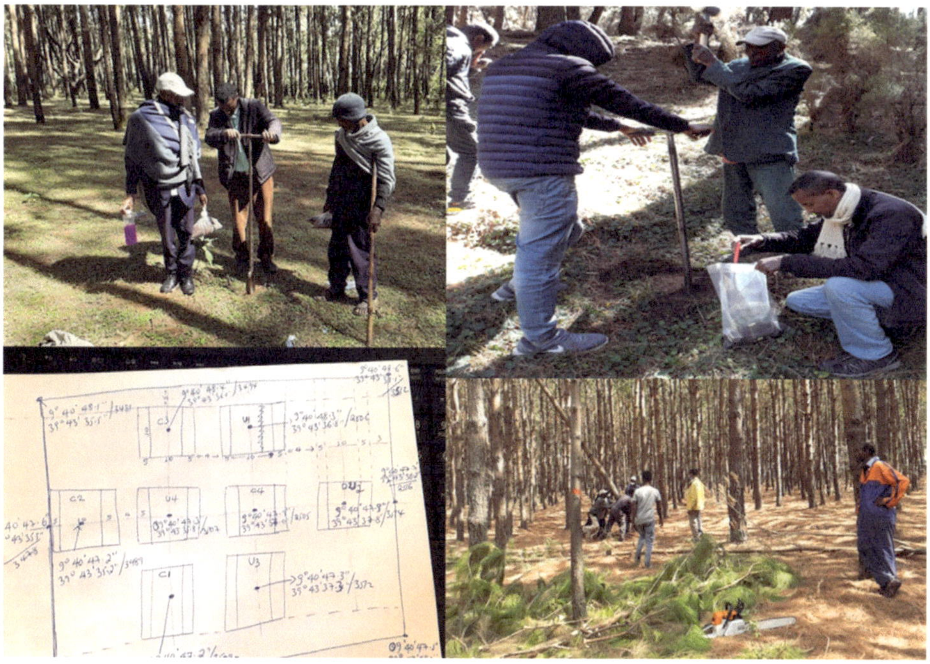

Figure 5.
Comprehensive studies of soil fungal community composition as a tool for sustainable conservation management. The photos depict various stages of research and field soil sampling, illustrating how these studies can inform effective management plans for preserving both forest and mycological resources within forest ecosystems.

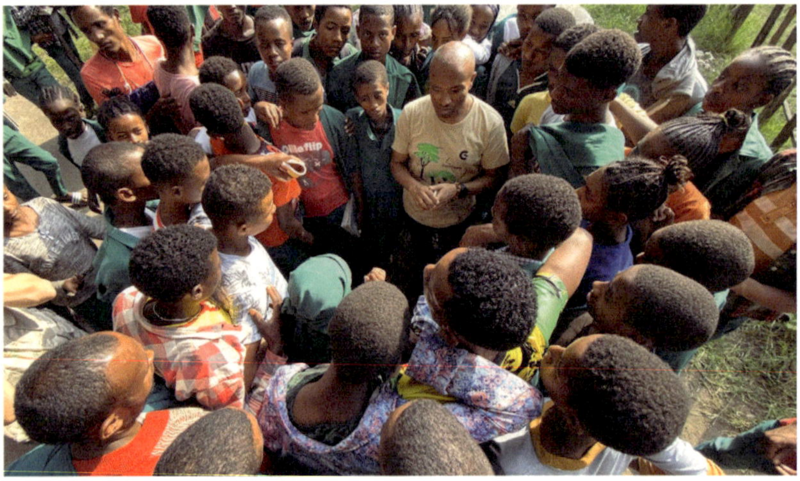

Figure 6.
A senior mycologist, coauthor of this work, educates youths about mushrooms and environmental education. The photo captures an engaging session where young learners are introduced to mushrooms and the importance of environmental stewardship.

decreasing their susceptibility to pests and diseases. This approach helps prevent tree mortality and the subsequent loss of associated resources, both timber and NTFPS, including economically and ecologically important mushrooms. Forest managers should prioritize mixed-species plantations and maintain diverse tree ages and sizes to create robust ecosystems. Additionally, implementing measures, such as controlled burns and thinning, can reduce competition for water and nutrients, further supporting tree health. Protecting and promoting fungal diversity through conservation efforts and habitat preservation is also vital, as fungi play a key role in nutrient cycling and soil health. Education and collaboration with local communities can ensure that sustainable practices are widely adopted, benefiting both the environment and the economy. By taking these steps, we can create forest ecosystems that are more resilient to climate change and continue to support valuable fungal communities.

Finally, the conservation of mushrooms through sustainable harvesting, farming, and management practices is essential to preserve their contribution to the environment and the economy. Ethiopia boasts a significant number of untapped wild mushrooms that are valuable sources of nutritional and medicinal value [61]. Research on the identification and preservation of these mushrooms, as illustrated in **Figure 5**, can contribute significantly to sustainable forest management and the conservation of mycological resources, avoiding overexploitation of this appreciated resource [9, 18, 49, 62]. As indicated in **Figure 6**, education and awareness-raising training on the importance of mushrooms and sustainable mushroom farming practices are essential for promoting their conservation and utilization [63].

6. Conclusion, implications, and future research directions

This chapter provides a comprehensive synthesis of the current state distribution and diversity of fungal species, the threats they face, and prospects for their conservation across various land uses (mainly forest stands) and sites in Ethiopia.

The results revealed a substantial diversity of fungal resources in Ethiopia. A high proportion of these edible species were found, which underscores the potential of Ethiopian forests as a source of wild edible mushrooms. However, it also highlights the need for careful management to ensure the sustainable use and conservation of these valuable resources. Considering their ecological roles (guilds), saprotrophic fungi were the dominant fungi, indicating their crucial role in nutrient cycling and decomposition processes within these forest ecosystems. The presence of ectomycorrhizal fungi further emphasizes the importance of symbiotic relationships in maintaining forest health and productivity.

As land use, land cover changes, deforestation, and climate change pose threats to the conservation of fungal diversity and their ecological functions, effective conservation strategies are essential. Understanding the distribution and ecological roles of fungi is crucial for developing these strategies. By identifying key fungal species and their habitats, management efforts can focus on protecting the most vulnerable and ecologically significant fungi, promoting the sustainable use of fungal resources in the country.

Overall, the implications of this study extend beyond academia to inform policy, practice, and public awareness efforts aimed at conserving fungal diversity and promoting sustainable forest management in Ethiopia (**Figure 7**). Therefore, it is important to take a multidisciplinary approach to fungal biodiversity, incorporating diverse perspectives to ensure the preservation and prosperity of this valuable resource for the benefit of both ecosystems and human communities. Future research should focus on further exploring unexplored habitats and utilizing advanced molecular techniques to uncover the hidden diversity of fungi. Continued efforts in fungal taxonomy, ecology, and conservation will enhance our understanding and contribute to the sustainable management of forest ecosystems.

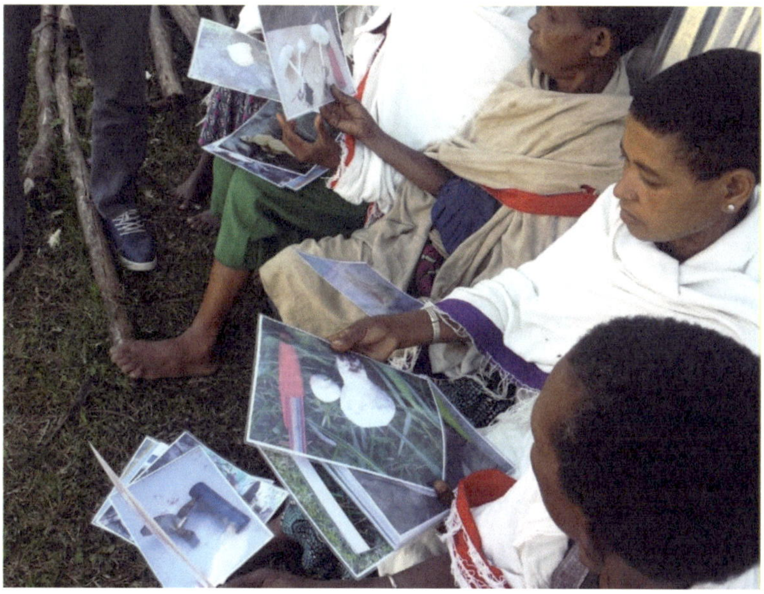

Figure 7.
The image shows training sessions, demonstrating common mushroom species for awareness creation among selected women's groups about ethnomycological knowledge on the use and conservation of mushrooms.

Conflict of interest

The authors declare no conflicts of interest.

Author details

Gonfa Kewessa[1,2], Tatek Dejene[3], Wubalem Tadesse[3] and Pablo Martín-Pinto[1*]

1 Sustainable Forest Management Research Institute, University of Valladolid, Avda. Madrid, Palencia, Spain

2 Department of Forestry, Ambo University, Ambo, Ethiopia

3 Ethiopian Forestry Development, Addis Ababa, Ethiopia

*Address all correspondence to: pmpinto@uva.es

References

[1] Hasan S, Gupta G. Fungal biodiversity: Evolution & distribution - A review. International Journal of Applied Research & Studies. 2012;**I**:1-8

[2] Antonelli A, Fry C, Smith RJ, Simmonds MSJ, Kersey PJ, Pritchard HW, et al. State of the World's Plants and Fungi 2020. London, England: Royal Botanic Garden; 2020. DOI: 10.34885/172

[3] Balami S, Vašutová M, Godbold D, Kotas P, Cudlín P. Soil fungal communities across land use types. iForest. 2020;**13**:548-558. DOI: 10.3832/ifor3231-013

[4] Manoharachary C, Sridhar K, Singh R, Adholeya A, Suryanarayanan TS, Rawat S, et al. Fungal biodiversity: Distribution, conservation and prospecting of fungi from India. Current Science. 2005;**89**:58-71

[5] Hawksworth DL, Lücking R. Fungal diversity revisited: 2.2 to 3.8 million species. The Fungal Kingdom. 2017;**89**(1):79-95. DOI: 10.1128/9781555819583.ch4

[6] Suryanarayanan TS, Hawksworth DL. Fungi from little-explored and extreme habitats. In: Deshmukh SK, Rai MK, editors. Biodivers Fungi their Role Hum Life. Enfield, USA: Science Publishers, Inc; 2005. pp. 33-48

[7] FAO. Global Forest Resources Assessment 2020. Main Report. Rome, Italy: FAO; 2020

[8] Higgins JPT, Altman DG, Gotzsche PC, Juni P, Moher D, Oxman AD, et al. The Cochrane collaboration's tool for assessing risk of bias in randomized trials. BMJ. 2011;**343**:d5928-d5928. DOI: 10.1136/bmj.d5928

[9] Alem D, Dejene T, Oria-De-rueda JA, Geml J, Martín-Pinto P. Soil fungal communities under *Pinus patula* Schiede ex Schltdl. & Cham. plantation forests of different ages in Ethiopia. Forests. 2020;**11**:1-18. DOI: 10.3390/f11101109

[10] Dejene T, Oria-de-Rueda JA, Martín-Pinto P. Fungal diversity and succession following stand development in *Pinus patula* Schiede ex Schltdl. & Cham. plantations in Ethiopia. Forest Ecology and Management. 2017;**395**:9-18. DOI: 10.1016/j.foreco.2017.03.032

[11] Castaño C, Dejene T, Mediavilla O, Geml J, Oria-de-Rueda JA, Martín-Pinto P. Changes in fungal diversity and composition along a chronosequence of *Eucalyptus grandis* plantations in Ethiopia. Fungal Ecology. 2019;**39**:328-335. DOI: 10.1016/j.funeco.2019.02.003

[12] Dejene T, Oria-de-Rueda JA, Martín-Pinto P. Fungal diversity and succession under *Eucalyptus grandis* plantations in Ethiopia. Forest Ecology and Management. 2017;**405**:179-187. DOI: 10.1016/j.foreco.2017.08.050

[13] Alem D, Dejene T, Oria-de-Rueda JA, Geml J, Castaño C, Smith JE, et al. Soil fungal communities and succession following wildfire in Ethiopian dry Afromontane forests, a highly diverse underexplored ecosystem. Forest Ecology and Management. 2020;**474**:118328. DOI: 10.1016/j.foreco.2020.118328

[14] Megersa S, Gure A, Feleke S, Alemu M. Macrofungi species richness and diversity in Dagaga and Gambo

plantation and natural forests of Arsi Forest Enterprise, Oromia, Ethiopia. Imperial Journal of Interdisciplinary Research. 2017;**3**:2454-1362. Available from: http://www.onlinejournal.in

[15] Alem D, Dejene T, Oria-de-Rueda JA, Martín-Pinto P. Survey of macrofungal diversity and analysis of edaphic factors influencing the fungal community of church forests in dry Afromontane areas of northern Ethiopia. Forest Ecology and Management. 2021;**496**:119391. DOI: 10.1016/j.foreco.2021.119391

[16] Alem D, Dejene T, Geml J, Oria-de-Rueda JA, Martín-Pinto P. Metabarcoding analysis of the soil fungal community to aid the conservation of underexplored church forests in Ethiopia. Scientific Reports. 2022;**12**:1-14. DOI: 10.1038/s41598-022-08828-3

[17] Sitotaw R, Mulat A, Abate D. Morphological and molecular studies on *Termitomyces* species of Menge District. Asossa zone, Northwest Ethiopia. Science, Technology and Arts Research Journal. 2016;**4**:49. DOI: 10.4314/star.v4i4.7

[18] Sitotaw R, Lulekal E, Abate D. Ethnomycological study of edible and medicinal mushrooms in Menge District, Asossa zone, Benshangul Gumuz region, Ethiopia. Journal of Ethnobiology and Ethnomedicine. 2020;**16**:1-14. DOI: 10.1186/s13002-020-00361-9

[19] Kewessa G, Dejene T, Alem D, Tolera M, Martín-Pinto P. Forest type and site conditions influence the diversity and biomass of edible *Macrofungal* species in Ethiopia. Journal of Fungi. 2022;**8**:1023. DOI: 10.3390/jof8101023

[20] Dejene T, Worku E, Martín-Pinto P. Retention of matured trees to conserve fungal diversity and edible sporocarps from short-rotation pinus radiata plantations in Ethiopia. Journal of Fungi. 2021;**7**:1-20. DOI: 10.3390/jof7090702

[21] Sitotaw R, Li Y, Wei TZ, Abate D, Yao YJ. Two new records of Agaricus spp. from Ethiopia. Mycotaxon. 2015;**130**:1171-1183. DOI: 10.5248/130.1171

[22] Wasihun P, Doda D. Study on prevalence and identification of ticks in Humbo district, southern nations, nationalities, and people's region (SNNPR), Ethiopia. Journal of Veterinary Medicine and Animal Health. 2013;**5**:73-80. DOI: 10.5897/JVMAH12.040

[23] Dejene T, Oria-de-Rueda JA, Martín-Pinto P. Wild mushrooms in Ethiopia: A review and synthesis for future perspective. Forestry Systems. 2017;**26**:eR02. DOI: 10.5424/fs/2017261-10790

[24] Geyid A, Abebe D, Debella A, Makonnen Z, Aberra F, Teka F, et al. Screening of some medicinal plants of Ethiopia for their antimicrobial properties and chemical profiles. Journal of Ethnopharmacology. 2005;**97**:421-427. DOI: 10.1016/j.jep.2004.08.021

[25] Mekuria Tadesse M, Alemu D, Abate N, Nigussie T, Zegeye S, Megersa B, et al. Atlas of Mushrooms:Global Versus Ethiopia. 1st ed. Vol. I. Ethiopia: Addis Ababa; 2023

[26] Dejene T, Oria-de-Rueda JA, Martín-Pinto P. Fungal community succession and sporocarp production following fire occurrence in dry Afromontane forests of Ethiopia. Forest Ecology and Management. 2017;**398**:37-47. DOI: 10.1016/j.foreco.2017.05.011

[27] Kewessa G, Dejene T, Martín-pinto P. Assessing the potential of

forest stands for edible mushrooms productivity as a subsistence ecosystem service in Ethiopia. Scientific African. 2023;**22**:e01936. DOI: 10.1016/j.sciaf.2023.e01936

[28] Tedersoo L, Bahram M, Dickie IA, et al. Does host plant richness explain diversity of ectomycorrhizal fungi? Re-evaluation of Gao datasets reveals sampling effects. Molecular Ecology. 2013;**23**(2014):992-995. DOI: 10.1111/mec.12660

[29] Tervonen K, Oldén A, Halme P. Ectomycorrhizal fungi in wood-pastures: Communities are determined by trees and soil properties, not by grazing. Agriculture, Ecosystems and Environment. 2019;**269**:13-21. DOI: 10.1016/j.agee.2018.09.015

[30] Wubet T, Kottke I, Teketay D, Oberwinkler F. Arbuscular mycorrhizal fungal community structures differ between co-occurring tree species of dry Afromontane tropical forest, and their seedlings exhibit potential to trap isolates suited for reforestation. Mycological Progress. 2009;**8**:317-328. DOI: 10.1007/s11557-009-0602-8

[31] Wu YT, Wubet T, Trogisch S, Both S, Scholten T, Bruelheide H, et al. Forest age and plant species composition determine the soil fungal community composition in a Chinese subtropical Forest. PLoS One. 2013;**8**:1-12. DOI: 10.1371/journal.pone.0066829

[32] Wubet T, Kottke I, Teketay D, Oberwinkler F. Mycorrhizal status of indigenous trees in dry Afromontane forests of Ethiopia. Forest Ecology and Management. 2003;**179**:387-399. DOI: 10.1016/S0378-1127(02)00546-7

[33] Shi Z, Yin K, Wang F, Mickan BS, Wang X, Zhou W, et al. Alterations of arbuscular mycorrhizal fungal diversity in soil with elevation in tropical forests of China. Diversity. 2019;**11**:1-10. DOI: 10.3390/d11100181

[34] Lilleskov EA, Fahey TJ, Horton TR, Lovett GM. Belowground ectomycorrhizal fungal community change over a nitrogen deposition gradient in Alaska. Ecology. 2002;**83**:104-115. DOI: 10.1890/0012-9658(2002)083(0104:BEFCCO)2.0.CO;2

[35] Treseder KK. A meta-analysis of mycorrhizal responses to nitrogen, phosphorus, and atmospheric CO_2 in field studies. The New Phytologist. 2004;**164**:347-355. DOI: 10.1111/j.1469-8137.2004.01159.x

[36] Wubet T, Weiß M, Kottke I, Teketay D, Oberwinkler F. Molecular diversity of arbuscular mycorrhizal fungi in *Prunus africana*, an endangered medicinal tree species in dry Afromontane forests of Ethiopia. The New Phytologist. 2004;**161**:517-528. DOI: 10.1046/j.1469-8137.2003.00924.x

[37] Mediavilla O, Oria-de-Rueda JA, Martín-Pinto P. Changes in sporocarp production and vegetation following wildfire in a Mediterranean forest ecosystem dominated by *Pinus nigra* in Northern Spain. Forest Ecology and Management. 2014;**331**:85-92. DOI: 10.1016/j.foreco.2014.07.033

[38] Janowski D, Leski T. Methods for identifying and measuring the diversity of ectomycorrhizal fungi. Forestry: An International Journal of Forest Research. 2023;**96**(5):1-14

[39] Wagg C, Jansa J, Stadler M, Schmid B, Van Der Heijden MGA. Mycorrhizal fungal identity and diversity relaxes plant–plant competition. Ecology. 2011;**92**:1303-1313. DOI: 10.1890/10-1915.1

[40] Nehls U. Mastering ectomycorrhizal symbiosis: The impact of carbohydrates. Journal of Experimental Botany. 2008;**59**:1097-1108. DOI: 10.1093/jxb/erm334

[41] Bonet JA, Fischer CR, Colinas C. The relationship between forest age and aspect on the production of sporocarps of ectomycorrhizal fungi in *Pinus sylvestris* forests of the Central Pyrenees. Forest Ecology and Management. 2004;**203**:157-175. DOI: 10.1016/j.foreco.2004.07.063

[42] Brown N, Bhagwat S, Watkinson S, Brown N, Bhagwatt S, Watkinson S. Macrofungal diversity in fragmented and disturbed forests of the Western Ghats of India. Journal of Applied Ecology. Feb 2006;**43**(1):11-17. DOI: 10.1111/j.1365-2664.2005.01107.x

[43] Boa E. Wild edible fungi: A global overview of their use and importance to people. Nonwood Forest Products. 2004;**17**:11-17. DOI: 10.1663/0013-0001(2006)60(99:wefago)2.0.co;2

[44] Adhikari MK, Devkota S, Tiwari RD. Ethnomycolgical knowledge on uses of wild mushrooms in Western and Central Nepal. Our Nature. 2006;**3**:13-19. DOI: 10.3126/on.v3i1.329

[45] Montoya A, Hernández-Totomoch O, Estrada-Torres A, Kong A, Caballero J. Traditional knowledge about mushrooms in a Nahua community in the state of Tlaxcala, México. Mycologia. 2003;**95**:793-806. DOI: 10.1080/15572536.2004.11833038

[46] Boa E. Wild edible fungi a global overview of their use and importance to people. Nonwood Forest Products (Rome, Italy: FAO). 2008;**17**

[47] Li H, Tian Y, Menolli N, Ye L, Karunarathna SC, Perez-Moreno J, et al. Reviewing the world's edible mushroom species: A new evidence-based classification system. Comprehensive Reviews in Food Science and Food Safety. 2021;**20**:1982-2014. DOI: 10.1111/1541-4337.12708

[48] Dejene T, Oria-de-Rueda JA, Martín-Pinto P. Edible wild mushrooms of Ethiopia: Neglected nontimber forest products. Revista Fitotecnia Mexicana. 2017;**40**:391-397. DOI: 10.35196/rfm.2017.4.391-397

[49] Zeleke G, Dejene T, Tadesse W, Agúndez D, Martín-Pinto P. Ethnomycological knowledge of three ethnic groups in Ethiopia. Forests. 2020;**11**:1-18. DOI: 10.3390/f11080875

[50] Shi L, Dossa GGO, Paudel E, Zang H, Xu J, Harrison RD. Changes in fungal communities across a forest disturbance gradient. BioRxiv. 2019;**85**:1-11. DOI: 10.1101/524132

[51] Teketay D. Deforestation, wood famine, and environmental degradation in Ethiopia's Highland ecosystems: Urgent need for action. Northeast African Studies. 2001;**8**:53-76. DOI: 10.1353/nas.2005.0020

[52] Coyle DR, Nagendra UJ, Taylor MK, Campbell JH, Cunard CE, Joslin AH, et al. Soil fauna responses to natural disturbances, invasive species, and global climate change: Current state of the science and a call to action. Soil Biology and Biochemistry. 2017;**110**:116-133. DOI: 10.1016/j.soilbio.2017.03.008

[53] Palit K, Rath S, Chatterjee S, et al. Microbial diversity and ecological interactions of microorganisms in the mangrove ecosystem: Threats, vulnerability, and adaptations. Environmental Science and Pollution Research. 2022;**29**:32467-32512. DOI: 10.1007/s11356-022-19048-7

[54] Damtie D, Mekonnen Y. Thymus species in Ethiopia: Distribution, medicinal value, economic benefit, current status and threatening factors. Ethiopian Journal of Science and Technology. 2015;**8**:81-92

[55] Mohammadi K, Khalesro S, Sohrabi Y, Heidari G, Review A. Beneficial effects of the Mycorrhizal fungi for plant growth. Journal of Applied Environmental and Biological Sciences. 2011;**1**:310-319

[56] Zhang Y, Dong S, Gao Q, Liu S, Ganjurjav H, Wang X, et al. Soil bacterial and fungal diversity differently correlated with soil biochemistry in alpine grassland ecosystems in response to environmental changes. Scientific Reports. 2017;7:1-10. DOI: 10.1038/srep43077

[57] Klestadt Laurindo L, de Souza TAF, da Silva LJR, dos Santos Nascimento G, da Cruz SP. *Pinus taeda* L changes arbuscular mycorrhizal fungi communities in a Brazilian subtropical ecosystem. Symbiosis. 2022;**87**:269-279. DOI: 10.1007/s13199-022-00875-8

[58] Weithmann G. Adjustment of hydraulic, anatomical and leaf traits in *Fagus sylvatica* (L.) toward drier conditions. A study in mature stands [Doctoral thesis]. Göttingen: Georg-August-University; 2022. p. 156. DOI: 10.53846/goediss-9409

[59] Bruns TD. Thoughts on the processes that maintain local species diversity of ectomycorrhizal fungi. In: Significance Regul Soil Biodivers. Netherlands: Springer; 1995. pp. 63-73. DOI: 10.1007/978-94-011-0479-1_5

[60] Nnadi NE, Carter DA. Climate change and the emergence of fungal pathogens. PLoS Pathogens. 2021;**17**:e1009503. DOI: 10.1371/journal.ppat.1009503

[61] Gizaw B. Traditional knowledge on mushroom consumption habits of Amhara region in four selected districts – Mecha, Fogera, Bahirdarzuria and Zege. Current Investigations in Agriculture and Current Research. 2018;**1**:11-18. DOI: 10.32474/ciacr.2018.01.000104

[62] Agúndez D, Tadesse W, Dejene T, Martín-Pinto P, Soliño M. Wild mushroom potential in Ethiopia: An analysis based on supplier and consumer preferences. Forestry Systems. 2022;**31**:e006. DOI: 10.5424/fs/2022312-18934

[63] Fernandes T, Garrine C, Ferrão J, Bell V, Varzakas T. Mushroom nutrition as preventative healthcare in sub-Saharan Africa. Applied Sciences. 2021;**11**(9):4221. DOI: 10.3390/app11094221

Chapter 2

Fungi Associated with Other Organisms: Diversity, Interactions and Ecological Importance

Laura Amália Miranda Costa, Flavia Helena Aires Sousa, Evelise Leis Carvalho, Fernando Augusto Bertazzo-Silva, Jorge Renato Pinheiro Velloso, Marcos André Pinheiro Velloso, Caio Henrique Lopes, Vanielle Galiano, Ana Flávia Zorzi, Ana Luiza Klotz-Neves and Jair Putzke

Abstract

Fungi play pivotal roles in ecosystems by forming diverse associations with other organisms, including plants, animals and microorganisms, along with certain bacteria. These interactions range from mutualistic relationships, such as mycorrhizal associations facilitating nutrient uptake in plants, to parasitic interactions causing disease in the hosts. Fungi also engage in commensal relationships, where one organism benefits without harming or significantly benefiting the other. The ecological importance of these associations is profound, influencing nutrient cycling, biodiversity, and ecosystem stability. For instance, lichens, composed of fungi and algae or cyanobacteria, are pioneer species in harsh environments and contribute to soil formation. Understanding the dynamics of fungal interactions with other organisms is crucial for ecosystem management and conservation efforts. Moreover, exploring the molecular mechanisms underlying these associations can offer insights into biotechnological applications, such as agriculture and medicine, harnessing the potential of fungi for sustainable solutions in various fields.

Keywords: symbiosis, maintaining biodiversity, nutrient cycling, biocontrol agents, ecological niches

1. Introduction

The understanding of the importance of fungi for both humans and the environment is only beginning to be explored, given their vast diversity and the challenges associated with studying their biology and ecology. Clearly defining the boundaries of an individual fungal species is a challenging task, as it is estimated that there are between 1.5 and 13.2 million species (based on different approaches) distributed across a wide variety of ecosystems known as mycobiomes [1–3].

These sites, also known as fungal communities, often exhibit a predominance of three main phyla: Ascomycota, Basidiomycota, and Chytridiomycota in aquatics environments, while in terrestrial ecosystems, it is common to find a predominance of the Ascomycota, Basidiomycota, and Zygomycota phylum [4–6]. Despite being a highly diverse group, these organisms interact with each other, with plants, and with animals to maintain the functional organization of their components [7].

Moreover, approximately 72–80% of all angiosperms outsource, at least partially, nutrient absorption, establishing a symbiotic relationship with arbuscular mycorrhizal (AM) fungi belonging to the subphylum Glomeromycotina [8, 9]. These fungi play a crucial role in nutrient uptake by plants. Free-living saprotrophic microorganisms are the primary agents responsible for decomposing soil organic matter, releasing essential nutrients for plant growth through the secretion of extracellular enzymes [10]. These close interactions between fungi and other organisms are essential for soil health and fertility.

The ecological interactions between fungi and other organisms play a fundamental role in the functionality of life on the planet. One of the greatest concerns among scientists is the extensive use of chemical substances, like pesticides, which can disrupt ecosystems and lead to soil and water contamination, as well as harm nontarget species [11].

An emerging and promising approach in agriculture for the control of nematodes, plants, and insect pests is the use of fungi. This alternative offers a viable and sustainable approach, regulating and naturally controlling pest populations [12]. For instance, over 700 species of fungi inhabiting the soil rhizosphere specialize in the biological control of nematodes [13].

Fungi also play important roles as pathogens, commensals, and mutualists of macroeukaryotic hosts. They pose challenges comparable to or even greater than other disease-causing agents: Currently, no vaccines are available for fungal pathogens, the arsenal of antifungal medications is extremely limited, and fungi can persist saprotrophically, releasing considerable amounts of infectious spores without requiring direct contact between hosts to initiate infection [14].

The characteristics of fungi and their ecological context, along with their interactions with other organisms, likely played a crucial role in ecosystem, ecological, and evolutionary processes, operating across various scales of time, space, and biological interactions. Increasing evidence suggests that fungi can facilitate connections among a wide range of organisms and ecosystems, potentially influencing the ecological, evolutionary, and biogeographic dynamics of associated organisms [15].

In this context, this chapter will explore a synthesis of interactions between fungi and other organisms, providing an updated review of related aspects, as well as future perspectives and challenges regarding these relationships.

2. Symbiotic fungi: Mycorrhizae and lichens

In most ecosystems, plants establish complex symbiotic relationships with other organisms, such as bacteria and fungi, which significantly influence development, promoting, or inhibiting growth. These relationships involve biochemical exchanges at the cellular level that affect plant physiology and have evolutionary implications, including species diversification, horizontal gene transfer, symbiosis, and mutualism. They also contribute to environmental adaptation and have positive impacts on community structure and biodiversity [16].

Among these relationships, the associations formed between terrestrial plants and mycorrhizal fungi are among the most crucial symbioses on Earth. Present in virtually all terrestrial ecosystems, from deserts and tropical forests to savannas and arable lands, these associations involve over 80% of terrestrial plant species, approximately 250,000 species, forming symbiotic associations with mycorrhizal fungi. These associations are vital for soil structure, nutrient cycling, plant diversity, and ecosystem sustainability [17, 18].

Mycorrhizal symbiosis is foundational for the diversity and existence of numerous fungal and plant species. Mycorrhizal fungi constitute a diverse group of soil fungi distinguished by their ability to form associations with plant roots. These subterranean fungi inhabit the cortex of plant roots, reside on the root surface, or surround the root epidermal cells. A vast network of fungal hyphae interconnects vegetation, ensuring nutrient distribution and tree sustenance. While some trees form associations with specific fungi, the role of fungi extends beyond these individual relationships to include the organization of plant communities and soil structure [19, 20].

The nutrient cycling driven by fungi is crucial for energy return to the soil, fostering the growth of new organisms and preventing the accumulation of undecomposed organic matter, thus avoiding energy stagnation [21]. Based on their structure and function, mycorrhizal symbioses are classified into four main types: arbuscular mycorrhiza, ectomycorrhiza, orchid mycorrhiza, and ericoid mycorrhiza [17].

Arbuscular mycorrhizae involve fungi from the phylum Glomeromycetes colonizing the roots of 80% of plant species, forming intracellular structures like arbuscules or coils. Ectomycorrhizal symbiosis occurs between plants and Basidiomycota, Ascomycota, and more rarely Zygomycota fungi, forming a hyphal sheath around the root tips, penetrating the intercellular space, and forming a network among cortical cells known as the Hartig net. This association is mainly observed in trees dominant in boreal, Mediterranean, temperate regions, and some tropical forests. In orchid and ericoid mycorrhizae, fungi form hyphal coils within the root cells of orchid species and plants of the *Ericaceae* family, respectively [22].

While orchid mycorrhizae are present in most *Orchidaceae* species, accounting for 10% of vascular plant species [23], ericoid mycorrhizae, found in some Ericaceae species, represent only 1.5% of vascular plants. Despite the relatively low plant diversity, ericoid mycorrhizae are present in various ecosystems, such as Mediterranean forests, tropical forests, and sandy plains, playing a key role in the soil carbon cycle [22].

Mycorrhizal fungi significantly influence plant productivity and diversity by connecting them below ground through a network of hyphae, allowing the movement of resources between coexisting plants. Moreover, symbiosis plays a fundamental role in the carbon, nitrogen, and phosphorus cycling in ecosystems [16]. Like mycorrhizal associations, lichenized fungi are one of the great examples of terrestrial symbiosis. A lichen constitutes a complex ecosystem formed through the interaction of a fungus (the mycobiont host), one or more photosynthetic partners (photobionts), and various other microscopic organisms such as bacteria and yeasts [24].

In this symbiosis, algae or cyanobacteria serve as photobionts, providing carbohydrates through photosynthesis, while the mycobiont host offers protection against desiccation. Additionally, cyanobacterial partners, known as cyanobionts, play a role in atmospheric nitrogen fixation [25].

Lichenized fungal forms evolved independently among Ascomycota and Basidiomycota; however, most lichen diversity is found in *Lecanoromycetes* and *Eurodiomycetes*. In contrast, the algal partners of most lichens belong to the phylum *Chlorophyta* and are largely dominated by *Trebouxiales* and *Trentepohliales* and, in a few known cases, *Ochrophyta* or streptophyte algae [26].

Lichens thrive in virtually all terrestrial ecosystems, surviving in extreme environments characterized by dryness, cold temperatures, or limited nutrient availability. They can colonize diverse surfaces, including rocks, soil, and tree bark, often forming biocrusts or growing as epiphytes. With an estimated species count of around 18,000, lichen diversity is particularly high in high-latitude regions, surpassing the species richness of vascular plants. Lichens perform multiple functions in the ecosystem, serving as food for reindeer and caribou, having a major role on the energy budget and albedo, and as biological indicators of atmospheric pollution [27].

In the last two decades, countless studies have attempted to elucidate the reasons behind and mechanisms of interactions among fungi and other organisms in the environment, with these interactions being crucial for the nutrient cycle and maintaining ecosystem balance [16].

When examining the complex beneficial interactions between organisms and fungi, one finds a diverse and ever-changing landscape that requires continued research in order to identify knowledge gaps and propose future directions for the investigation of fungal symbionts.

3. Endophytic fungi

The interaction between plants and microorganisms in natural ecosystems significantly influences plant growth, development, and defensive capabilities against biotic stresses and potential threats posed by other organisms [28]. Among the myriad of observed interactions, particular attention is given to the symbiotic relationship between plants and endophytic fungi, a notably diverse group estimated to encompass up to 3.1 million species [29].

These organisms colonize the internal tissues of plants during various stages of their life cycles without causing harm to the host plant under any circumstances [30]. The assembly of endophytic fungal communities is directly influenced by the environmental conditions within the plant's habitat, leading to variations in endophytic fungal species even within the same plant species across different locations [31, 32].

The intricate relationship between endophytes and their host plants is highlighted by the capacity of these fungi to produce secondary metabolites that closely resemble those synthesized by the host plants themselves [33]. Moreover, these fungi positively influence the biogeochemical cycles of plants, thereby impacting processes such as photosynthesis [34].

This observation of chemotactic signaling in endophytic interactions suggests that these microorganisms are not mere opportunists but rather products of coevolutionary adaptations between species [35]. Fossil records indicate that the association between plants and endophytes, as well as mycorrhizae, dates back 400 million years, coinciding with the colonization of soil by plants. This underscores the significance of this association in the evolutionary process of these organisms [36, 37].

This coevolutionary relationship has driven the development of genetic traits in these organisms to ensure mutual survival, leading to the emergence of biochemical mechanisms against pathogenic agents [38, 39]. The association between endophytic fungi and plants is mutualistic, fostering beneficial processes for both parties involved. In this context, while the plant provides a habitat for survival, the fungal partner assumes a biostimulant role, producing bioactive compounds essential for the plant's growth and survival [40].

Recent investigations have identified various endophytic fungi in Tartary buckwheat (*Fagopyrum tataricum* (L.) Gaertn.) and established correlations between their presence and the production of flavonoids in the plant, indicating enhancements in the medicinal properties of the crop. Additionally, researchers have observed the influence of endophytic fungi on the phenotypic characteristics of plants, suggesting a potential association between fungal symbiosis and plant growth traits [41].

Different endophytic fungi have exhibited varying impacts on the growth and metabolism of *Salvia miltiorrhiza* Bunge., enhancing the net photosynthetic rate, intercellular CO_2 concentration, and crucial enzymatic activities. Moreover, these fungi have improved the plant's adaptability and resistance to environmental stresses by increasing the synthesis of osmoregulatory compounds and enhancing enzymatic antioxidant activity [42].

Diversified *in situ* and *in vitro* analyses have been utilized to explore the effects of endophytic fungi on plants and their influence on associated biological processes [43, 44]. The insights obtained not only contribute valuable knowledge to our understanding of the biology of this symbiotic relationship and the ecology of these organisms but also lay the groundwork for novel discoveries and biotechnological applications.

The dissemination of these findings not only facilitates the sharing of scientific knowledge but also catalyzes research endeavors aimed at bioprospecting and leveraging the potential of these organisms for diverse biotechnological processes.

4. Fungi as bioindicators and biocontrol agents

Fungi are significant producers of secondary metabolites and can exhibit antibiotic, insecticidal, and immunosuppressive activities, with potential medicinal or known microbial agent properties. These properties and activities have been studied on a large scale in many areas [45].

These characteristics can prove valuable in implementing processes such as the remediation of pesticides, which are often applied in large quantities and contribute to soil and water contamination. Synthetic and anthropogenic substances are closely associated with environmental pollution, and the application of pesticides can lead to harmful alterations in entomopathogenic fungi (EPF) which have beneficial actions in the Integrated Pest Management (IPM) program [46].

Brazil is a major producer of crops such as soybeans and has witnessed rapid growth in the utilization of entomopathogenic fungi (EPF) as biopesticides over the past 5 years. There is significant interest in adapting bioproducts for large-scale distribution to meet consumer demand. These products aim to promote plant growth, facilitate the establishment of agroecosystems, and reduce the application of chemical pesticides [47, 48].

Despite the availability of information, only a few fungal genera have had their potential evaluated for controlling agricultural pests and practical applications in the world. Many species remain unexplored due to the scarcity of research involving endophytic fungi and entomopathogenic fungi (EPF). The genera *Beauveria*, *Metarhizium*, *Lecanicillium*, and *Cordyceps* (formerly *Isaria*) are the most commonly utilized in the formulation of fungal-based products for combating pests during cultivation and the postharvest period of agricultural products [49].

There is a growing demand for a better understanding of the host recognition process of EPF to produce more effective and specific biocontrol agents. Insects' adaptive reactions can be influenced by climate change, leading to alterations in the immune and physiological responses of the group. EPF typically exhibits negligible performance at temperatures close to 37°C [50, 51]. They develop adhesive structures that enhance penetration of the insect cuticle, particularly in species such as ants, termites, and flies. These insects are capable of self-cleaning to eliminate the parasite's spores [52–54].

The development and enhancement of new, more sustainable agricultural techniques and practices involving molecular mechanisms are necessary to reinforce plant resistance and increase crop resilience. The occurrence of a disease in a plant depends on three factors: organism susceptibility, the presence of virulent pathogens, and appropriate environmental conditions. This correlation is often referred to as the 'disease triangle' [55, 56].

Fungi exhibit a high sensitivity to changes in the ecosystem, making them valuable indicators of environmental shifts and subjects of study. While research on the use of microorganisms as bioindicators has expanded significantly in recent years, information specifically on fungal indicators remains relatively scarce [57].

Understanding these processes is crucial for harnessing and utilizing EPF as an effective biocontrol agent. EPF can also play a role in the production of nanoparticles (AgNPs). The biosynthesis of AgNPs offers various applications with antibacterial and antifungal properties, which can be achieved through enzymes present in the environment. These particles have demonstrated effectiveness in controlling diseases transmitted by vectors, addressing significant concerns for public health. As global temperatures continue to rise, modifications in the fungal life cycle may influence the emergence of more prevalent disease outbreaks [46, 50].

In addition to insects, nematodes represent another predominant group involved in interactions with fungi, often coexisting in a wide range of habitats. This relationship is termed as a 'tripartite interaction'. In these interactions, plant pathogens and pests frequently occupy the same space, engaging in synergistic exchanges and chemical signaling. The mode of action of pathogenic agents is influenced by physiological conditions. Nematodes can reduce plant resistance and inflict significant damage and losses [58].

Nematophagous fungi (NTF) are recognized for their ability to capture and kill nematodes through specific structures. The refinement of these structures and the development of countermeasures against nematodes are influenced by both biotic factors (such as microbes and plants) and abiotic factors (including nutrient availability). They also demonstrate higher effectiveness in biological control compared to bacteria and viruses, particularly in combating plant parasites. Understanding biotrophic interactions between NTF and nematodes is essential for elucidating the functioning of ecological niches and processes such as nutrient cycling and matter decomposition [58–60].

The mechanism of action and predatory activity of fungi shows a high degree of specificity. They are capable of releasing or producing enzymes, biochemical properties, and certain biotic and abiotic factors that can grow on any insect. The relationship between fungi and other organisms has several benefits. The analysis of these associations can help in the management of biodiversity. Thus, alternatives for the use of more sustainable, effective, and efficient chemicals can be found in many agricultural areas worldwide.

5. Saprotrophic fungi as decomposers

Saprotrophic fungi are those that decompose organic matter, enabling the cycling of nutrients in ecosystems. These organisms continuously deplete resources in the environment, and therefore their success depends on their ability to spread to new food sources, exclusively through the production of propagules (spores or hyphal fragments), given that in terrestrial environments, resources are distributed heterogeneously in space and time [61, 62].

Another factor of great importance for the colonization and establishment of saprotrophic fungi relates to their enzymatic capacity. If the fungus has the enzymatic potential to utilize the compounds available in the resource, it will colonize, establish, and persist until being displaced by another species, inhibited, or killed by adverse abiotic conditions, or until the food supply is exhausted [63].

When considering saprotrophic fungi, Basidiomycota stand out, including the causes of brown rot and white rot, presenting their own enzymatic characteristics regarding the deterioration of the substrate's chemical components. The former decomposes the polysaccharides of the cell wall, and the attacked wood shows a brown coloration. The latter decomposes both polysaccharides and lignin, and the wood shows a more white-like appearance [64].

During the decomposition process of organic matter, it is known that saprotrophic fungi are capable of producing methane, being considered important emitters of this gas into the atmosphere, not just carbon dioxide. Some studies have even shown that there is an association between this ecological group of fungi and methanogenic Archaea, which use this CH4 as their food source [65].

Finally, understanding the relationships of saprotrophic fungi with other organisms present in a wide range of ecosystems is of paramount importance to clarify the true extent of their ecological role. Furthermore, categorizing the diversity of fungi in decomposers is an important issue that will help preserve soil quality and maximize the carbon storage capacity of these ecosystems [66].

6. Practical applications

Fungi play an indispensable role in the Earth's ecological balance, nutrient regulation, and biodiversity maintenance. In symbiotic relationships with plants, fungi are pivotal for the survival and longevity of trees by facilitating access to otherwise inaccessible nutrients [67]. Furthermore, the interdependence of fungi and plants not only preserves the biodiversity of plants in these environments but also supports ecosystem functionalities [68].

Fungi also plays a role in mitigating anthropogenic environmental impacts. They are involved in the remediation of environmental disasters, including soil degradation and pollution from toxic wastes and oil spills, facilitating the recovery and preservation of ecosystems [69–71]. The imperative to lessen human impact on nature has spurred interest in sustainable alternatives to fossil fuels. Fungi, such as those in the genus *Mucor*, are being investigated for their potential in biodiesel production due to their enzyme production capabilities and high lipid content [72].

Beyond environmental applications, fungi have significant economic value in the production of food, beverages, medicines, and bioenergy. For example, yeast is integral to the production of bread and alcoholic beverages through fermentation processes [73]. In the medical field, fungi are being explored for their therapeutic potential, such as the genus *Psilocybe* in treating depression [74]. Additionally, in veterinary medicine, fungi offer solutions for controlling diseases in livestock, such as nematode infestations in cattle, with the genus *Monacrosporium* providing biocontrol agents [75].

The diverse functionalities and applications of fungi underscore their crucial role in ecosystem maintenance, biodiversity, health, and economic activities. A better understanding of the microbiome and its relationships with different associations established with other genera and groups will help conserve fungi.

7. Conclusions

It is known that a significant portion of the interactions between plants and animals is related to fungi, and increasingly, research is uncovering associations that this group has in nature. There are numerous challenges in controlling the threats to the habitats of these organisms and conserving their interactions. Despite the proliferation of actions and campaigns aimed at preserving the environment and its resources, many individuals and large corporations persist in adopting inappropriate practices [76].

Climate change is one of the consequences of habitat loss, emerging as one of the most alarming factors when considering current and future challenges related to organisms associated with fungal groups. A significant portion of the diversity found in various regions worldwide comprises fungal associations. However, with advancements in science and mycology, coupled with the utilization of increasingly sophisticated techniques and cross-border collaborations, there are prospects for fungi to contribute to the restoration of spaces damaged by anthropogenic activities. This is owing to their functional potential within ecosystems, where they perform several essential life functions. The imperative to preserve forests and ecosystems reliant on biotic interactions for equilibrium is evident [77].

Consequently, the utilization of fungi emerges as a crucial conservation strategy, addressing issues such as air and water purification while mitigating diseases stemming from environmental transformations. Fungi not only aid in maintaining microclimates but also play a pivotal role in soil nutrient recycling and the nourishment of associated organisms. As for emerging fungal-related diseases, their proliferation is partially attributed to environmental degradation, which heightens the risk of incidence [78].

Some of the possible future reflections pertain to technological innovation aimed at further exploring fungal contributions to food production, the pharmaceutical industry, biodegradation processes, biological treatment of effluents, agricultural and ecological industries, biotransformation work, among others. All these areas, which have already been studied, may contribute even more to the new developments and advances that will be experienced in the future, manipulating fungi to obtain these new technologies for the benefit of society and the environment [79].

Additionally, their potential as bioindicators can be leveraged to elucidate areas where environmental imbalance exists, enabling the promotion of resolution that may even utilize fungi themselves and their associations for restoration and mitigation [80]. However, the study of fungi demands an interdisciplinary approach to prevent a narrow, reductionist perspective confined to isolated disciplines. Fungi exemplify transformative potentials, both in our comprehension of life and in fostering collective relationships.

It is important to highlight the fungi's capability to create extensive mycorrhizal networks that not only facilitate nutrient distribution but also enable communication across forest ecosystems, alerting them to biological threats. This organized, collective action of fungi, maintaining ecological equilibrium, serves as a model for human collaboration.

By emulating these fungal networks, humanity can enhance its approach to collective living and environmental stewardship, deepening our connection with the natural world and advancing our biotechnological endeavors through a more profound understanding of fungal processes and their integrative roles in Earth's biosphere.

Acknowledgements

We would like to thank the team of LATAF (Laboratório de Taxonomia de Fungos), of Universidade Federal do Pampa (UNIPAMPA) for the support of this research. This study was financed in part by the Coordenação de Aperfeiçoamento de Pessoal de Nível Superior – Brasil (CAPES) – Finance Code 001 and by Fundação de Amparo à Pesquisa do Estado do Rio Grande do Sul (FAPERGS) under nbr. 21/2551-0001985-9 and Conselho Nacional de Pesquisa (CNPQ) nbr. 405564/2022-8.

Conflict of interest

The authors declare no conflict of interest.

Author details

Laura Amália Miranda Costa[1], Flavia Helena Aires Sousa[1], Evelise Leis Carvalho[1], Fernando Augusto Bertazzo-Silva[1], Jorge Renato Pinheiro Velloso[1], Marcos André Pinheiro Velloso[1], Caio Henrique Lopes[2], Vanielle Galiano[2], Ana Flávia Zorzi[3], Ana Luiza Klotz-Neves[1] and Jair Putzke*

1 Programa de Pós-Graduação em Ciências Biológicas (PPGCB), Universidade Federal do Pampa, São Gabriel, Brazil

2 Universidade Federal do Pampa, São Gabriel, Brazil

3 Programa de Pós-Graduação em Educação em Ciências (PPgECi), Universidade Federal de Santa Maria, Santa Maria, Brazil

*Address all correspondence to: jrputzkebr@yahoo.com

References

[1] Hawksworth DL, Lücking R. Fungal diversity revisited: 2.2 to 3.8 million species. Microbiology Spectrum. 2017;**5**:10. DOI: 10.1128/microbiolspec.funk-0052-2016

[2] Wu B, Hussain M, Zhang W, Stadler M, Liu X, Xiang M. Current insights into fungal species diversity and perspective on naming the environmental DNA sequences of fungi. Mycology. 2019;**10**:127-140. DOI: 10.1080/21501203.2019.1614106

[3] Tedersoo L, Mikryukov V, Anslan S, et al. The global soil mycobiome consortium dataset for boosting fungal diversity research. Fungal Diversity. 2021;**111**:573-588. DOI: 10.1007/s13225-021-00493-7

[4] Hassett BT, Vonnahme TR, Peng X, Jones EBG, Heuzé C. Global diversity and geography of planktonic marine fungi. Botanica Marina. 2020;**63**:121-139. DOI: 10.1515/bot-2018-0113

[5] Tedersoo L, Bahram M, Põlme S, Kõljalg U, Yorou NS, Wijesundera R, et al. Fungal biogeography. Global diversity and geography of soil fungi. Science. 2014;**346**(6213):1256688. DOI: 10.1126/science.1256688

[6] Naranjo-Ortiz MA, Gabaldón T. Fungal evolution: Diversity, taxonomy and phylogeny of the fungi. Biological Reviews. 2019;**94**(6):2101-2137

[7] Topalović O, Heuer H. Plant-nematode interactions assisted by microbes in the rhizosphere. Current Issues in Molecular Biology. 2019;**30**:75-88. DOI: 10.21775/cimb.030.075

[8] Brundrett MC, Tedersoo L. Evolutionary history of mycorrhizal symbioses and global host plant diversity. New Phytologist. 2018;**220**(4):1108-1115. DOI: 10.1111/nph.14976

[9] Spatafora JW, Chang Y, Benny GL, Lazarus K, Smith ME, Berbee ML, et al. A phylum-level phylogenetic classification of zygomycete fungi based on genome-scale. Mycologia. 2016;**108**(5):1028-1046. DOI: 10.3852/16-042

[10] Baldrian P. Forest microbiome: Diversity, complexity and dynamics. FEMS Microbiology Reviews. 2017;**41**(2):109-130. DOI: 10.1093/femsre/fuw040

[11] Inobeme A, Mathew JT, Okonkwo S, Al A, Jacob JO, Olori E. Pesticide residues in food: Distribution, route of exposure and toxicity: in review. MOJ Food Processing & Technology. 2020;**8**(3):121-124. DOI: 10.15406/mojfpt.2020.08.002516

[12] Savita SA. Fungi as biological control agents. In: Giri B, Prasad R, Wu QS, Varma A, editors. Biofertilizers for Sustainable Agriculture and Environment. Soil Biology. 55th ed. Cham, Switzerland: Springer; 2019. pp. 395-413. DOI: 10.1007/978-3-030-18933-4

[13] Jiang X, Xiang M, Liu X. Nematode-trapping fungi. Microbiology Spectrum. 2017;**5**(1):1-12. DOI: 10.1128/microbiolspec.funk-0022-2016

[14] Casadevall A. Global catastrophic threats from the fungal kingdom: Fungal catastrophic threats. Current Topics in Microbiology and Immunology. 2019;**424**:21-32. DOI: 10.1007/82_2019_161

[15] Bahram M, Netherway T. Fungi as mediators linking organisms and ecosystems. FEMS Microbiology Reviews. 2022;**46**(2):fuab058. DOI: 10.1093/femsre/fuab058

[16] Chiquito-Contreras CJ, Meza-Menchaca T, Guzmán-López O, Vásquez EC, Ricaño-Rodríguez J. Molecular insights into plant-microbe interactions: A comprehensive review of key mechanisms. Frontiers in Bioscience (Elite Edition). 2024;**16**(1):9. DOI: 10.31083/j.fbe1601009

[17] Martin FM, Heijden MGA. The mycorrhizal symbiosis: Research frontiers in genomics, ecology, and agricultural application. The New Phytologist. 2024;**242**:1486-1506. DOI: 10.1111/nph.19541

[18] Hawkins HJ, Cargill RIM, Van Nuland ME, Hagen SC, Field KJ, Sheldrake M, et al. Mycorrhizal mycelium as a global carbon pool. Current Biology. 2023;**33**(11):R560-R573. DOI: 10.1016/j.cub.2023.02.027

[19] Berbara Ricardo LL, Souza Francisco A, Fonseca HMAC. III-Fungos micorrízicos arbusculares: muito além da nutrição. In: Nutrição mineral de plantas. Viçosa, MG: Sociedade Brasileira de Ciência do Solo; 2006. pp. 74-85

[20] Berude M, Almeida D, Riva M, Cabanêz P, Amaral A. Micorrizas e sua importância agroecológica. Enciclopédia Biosfera. 2015;**11**(22):132-146

[21] Cavalcante FG, Bandeira LL, Leite LO, da Silva AO, de Mesquita AFN, de Matos Neto JM, et al. Grupos Funcionais do solo: papel das comunidades microbianas especializadas na ciclagem de nutrientes e sensores de distúrbios ambientais. Cuadernos de Educación y Desarrollo. 2023;**15**(9):8676-8698. DOI: 10.55905/cuadv15n9-038

[22] Mujica MI, Herrera H, Cisternas M, Zuniga-Feest A, Sagredo-Saez C, Selosse MA. Mycorrhizas in south American *Ericaceae*. Mycorrhiza. 2024;**34**:1-18. DOI: 10.1007/s00572-024-01141-z

[23] Selosse MA, Petrolli R, Mujica MI, Laurent L, Perez-Lamarque B, Figura T, et al. The waiting room hypothesis revisited by orchids: Were orchid mycorrhizal fungi recruited among root endophytes? Annals of Botany. 2022;**129**(3):259-270. DOI: 10.1093/aob/mcab134

[24] Hawksworth DL, Grube M. Lichens redefined as complex ecosystems. New Phytologist. 2020;**227**:1281-1283. DOI: 10.1111/nph.16630

[25] Rodríguez-Arribas C, Martínez I, AragónG,Zamorano-ElguetaC,CavieresL, Prieto M. Specialization patterns in symbiotic associations: A community perspective over spatial scales. Ecology and Evolution. 2023;**13**(7):e10296. DOI: 10.1002/ece3.10296

[26] Bonito G. Ecology and evolution of algal-fungal symbioses. Current Opinion in Microbiology. 2024;**79**:102452. DOI: 10.1016/j.mib.2024.102452

[27] Rautiainen M, Kuusinen N, Majasalmi T. Remote sensing and spectroscopy of lichens. Ecology and Evolution. 2024;**14**(3):e11110. DOI: 10.1002/ece3.11110

[28] Nataraja KN, Suryanarayanan TS, Shaanker RU, Senthil-Kumar M, Oelmüller R. Plant–microbe interaction: Prospects for crop improvement and management. Plant Physiology Reports. 2019;**24**:461-462. DOI: 10.1007/s40502-019-00494-4

[29] Bhunjun CS, Phukhamsakda C, Hyde KD, McKenzie EH, Saxena RK, Li Q. Do all fungi have ancestors with endophytic lifestyles? Fungal Diversity. 2024;**125**:73-98. DOI: 10.1007/s13225-023-00516-5

[30] Le Cocq K, Gurr SJ, Hirsch PR, Mauchline TH. Exploitation of endophytes for sustainable agricultural intensification. Molecular Plant Pathology. 2017;**18**(3):469-473. DOI: 10.1111/mpp.12483

[31] Vega FE, Simpkins A, Aime MC, Posada F, Peterson SW, Rehner SA, et al. Fungal endophyte diversity in coffee plants from Colombia, Hawaii, Mexico and Puerto Rico. Fungal Ecology. 2010;**3**(3):122-138. DOI: 10.1016/j.funeco.2009.07.002

[32] Aly AH, Debbab A, Proksch P. Fungal endophytes: Unique plant inhabitants with great promises. Applied Microbiology and Biotechnology. 2011;**90**(6):1829-1845. DOI: 10.1007/s00253-011-3270-y

[33] Tejesvi MV, Pirttilä AM. Endophytic fungi, occurrence, and metabolites. In: Anke T, Schüffler A, editors. Physiology and Genetics. Cham, Switzerland: Springer; 2018. pp. 213-230. DOI: 10.3390%2Fpathogens10050570

[34] Luo J, Liu T, Diao F, Hao B, Zhang Z, Hou Y, et al. Shift in rhizospheric and endophytic microbial communities of dominant plants around Sunit alkaline Lake. Science of the Total Environment. 2023;**867**:161503. DOI: 10.1016/j.scitotenv.2023.161503

[35] Schulz B, Boyle C. The endophytic continuum. Mycological Research. 2005;**109**:661-686. DOI: 10.1017/s095375620500273x

[36] Krings M, Taylor TN, Hass H, Kerp H, Dotzler N, Hermsen EJ. Fungal endophytes in a 400-million-yr-old land plant: Infection pathways, spatial distribution, and host responses. New Phytologist. 2007;**174**(3):648-657. DOI: 10.1111/j.1469-8137.2007.02008.x

[37] Rai M, Rathod D, Agarkar G, Dar M, Brestic M, Pastore GM, et al. Fungal growth promotor endophytes: A pragmatic approach towards sustainable food and agriculture. Symbiosis. 2014;**62**:63-79. DOI: 10.1007/s13199-014-0273-3

[38] Bielecka M, Pencakowski B, Nicoletti R. Using next-generation sequencing technology to explore genetic pathways in endophytic fungi in the syntheses of plant bioactive metabolites. Agriculture. 2022;**12**(2):187. DOI: 10.3390/agriculture12020187

[39] Usman M, Shah IH, Sabir IA, Malik MS, Rehman A, Murtaza G, et al. Synergistic partnerships of endophytic fungi for bioactive compound production and biotic stress management in medicinal plants. Plant Stress. 2024;**11**(2):100425. DOI: 10.1016/j.stress.2024.100425

[40] Rustamova N, Litao N, Bozorov K, Sayyed R, Aisa HA, Yili A. Plant-associated endophytic fungi: A source of structurally diverse and bioactive natural products. Plant Cell Biotechnology and Molecular Biology. 2022;**23**:1-19. DOI: 10.56557/pcbmb/2022/v23i7-87454

[41] Chen M, Ding Z, Zhou M, Shang Y, Li C, Li Q, et al. The diversity of endophytic fungi in Tartary buckwheat (*Fagopyrum tataricum*) and its correlation with flavonoids and phenotypic traits. Frontiers in Microbiology. 2024;**15**:1360988. DOI: 10.3389/fmicb.2024.1360988

[42] Li X, Lin Y, Qin Y, Han G, Wang H, Yan Z. Beneficial endophytic

fungi improve the yield and quality of *Salvia miltiorrhiza* by performing different ecological functions. PeerJ. 2024;**12**:e16959. DOI: 10.7717%2Fpeerj.16959

[43] Fontana DC, de Paula S, Torres AG, de Souza VHM, Pascholati SF, Schmidt D, et al. Endophytic fungi: Biological control and induced resistance to phytopathogens and abiotic stresses. Pathogens. 2021;**10**(5):570. DOI: 10.3390/pathogens10050570

[44] Wani ZA, Ashraf N, Mohiuddin T, Riyaz-Ul-Hassan S. Plant-endophyte symbiosis, an ecological perspective. Applied Microbiology and Biotechnology. 2015;**99**(7):2955-2965. DOI: 10.1007/s00253-015-6487-3

[45] Zhang L, Li S, Li H, Wang R, Zhang KQ, Xu J. Secondary metabolites from hypocrealean entomopathogenic fungi: Novel bioactive compounds. Natural Product Reports. 2020;**37**:1181-1206. DOI: 10.1039%2Fc9np00065h

[46] Litwin A, Nowak M, Różalska S. Entomopathogenic fungi: Unconventional applications. Reviews in Environmental Science and Biotechnology. 2020;**19**:23-42. DOI: 10.1007/s11157-020-09525-1

[47] CONAB - Brazilian National Food Supply Agency [Companhia Nacional do Abastecimento]. Acompanhamento da Safra Brasileira. Brasília-DF, Brazil: CONAB - Brazilian National Food Supply Agency [Companhia Nacional do Abastecimento]; 2022. Bol. da Safra, 2021. Available from: https://www.conab.gov.br/info-agro/safras/

[48] Faria M, Mascarin GM, Butt T, Lopes RB. On-farm production of microbial Entomopathogens for use in agriculture: Brazil as a case study. Neotropical Entomology. 2023;**52**:122-133. DOI: 10.1007/s13744-023-01033-5

[49] Bamisile BS, Afolabi OG, Siddiqui JA, Xu Y. Endophytic insect pathogenic fungi-host plant-herbivore mutualism: Elucidating the mechanisms involved in the tripartite interactions. World Journal of Microbiology and Biotechnology. 2023;**39**:326. DOI: 10.1007/s11274-023-03780-4

[50] St, Leger RJ. Insects and their pathogens in a changing climate. Journal of Invertebral Pathology. 2021;**184**:107644. DOI: 10.1016/j.jip.2021.107644

[51] Siscar-Lewin S, Hube B, Brunke S. Emergence and evolution of virulence in human pathogenic fungi. Trends in Microbiology. 2022;**30**:693-704. DOI: 10.1016/j.tim.2021.12.013

[52] Casillas-Pérez B, Boďová K, Grasse AV, Tkačik G, Cremer S. Dynamic pathogen detection and social feedback shape collective hygiene in ants. Nature Communications. 2023;**14**:3232. DOI: 10.1038/s41467-023-38947-y

[53] Shang J, Tang G, Yang J, Lu M, Wang CZ, Wang C. Sensing of a spore surface protein by a *Drosophila* chemosensory protein induces behavioral defense against fungal parasitic infections. Current Biology. 2023;**33**:276-286. DOI: 10.1016/j.cub.2022.11.004

[54] Hong S, Shang J, Sun Y, Tang G, Wang C. Fungal infection of insects: Molecular insights and prospects. Trends in Microbiology. 2024;**32**(3):302-316. DOI: 10.1016/j.tim.2023.09.005

[55] Waheed A, Haxim Y, Islam W, Ahmad M, Muhammad M, Alqahtani FM, et al. Climate change reshaping plant-fungal interaction. Environmental Research.

2023;**30**:117282. DOI: 10.1016/j.envres.2023.117282

[56] Liu Y, He F. Incorporating the disease triangle framework for testing the effect of soil-borne pathogens on tree species diversity. Functional Ecology. 2019;**33**:1211-1222. DOI: 10.1111/1365-2435.13345

[57] Warnasuriya SD, Udayanga DS, Biles MC. Fungi as environmental bioindicators. Science of the Total Environment. 2023;**892**:164583. DOI: 10.1016/j.scitotenv.2023.164583

[58] Zhang Y, Li S, Li H, Wang R, Zhang KQ, Xu J. Fungi–nematode interactions: Diversity, ecology, and biocontrol prospects in agriculture. Journal of Fungi. 2020;**6**:206. DOI: 10.3390/jof6040206

[59] Al-Ani LK, Soares FE, Sharma A, de Los S-VS, Valdivia-Padilla AV, Aguilar-Marcelino L. Strategy of nematophagous fungi in determining the activity of plant parasitic nematodes and their prospective role in sustainable agriculture. Frontiers in Fungal Biology. 2023;**3**:863198. DOI: 10.3389/ffunb.2022.863198

[60] Saeed M, Mukhtar T, Ahmed R, Ahmad T, Iqbal MA. Suppression of *Meloidogyne javanica* infection in peach (*Prunus persica* (L.) Batsch) using fungal biocontrol agents. Sustainability. 2023;**15**:13833. DOI: 10.3390/su151813833

[61] Boddy L. The microenvironment of basidiomycete mycelia in temperate deciduous woodlands. In: Jennings DH, Rayner ADM, editors. Ecology and Physiology of the Fungal Mycelium. Cambridge, United Kingdom: Cambridge University Press; 1984. pp. 261-289

[62] Boddy L. Saprotrophic cord-forming fungi: Meeting the challenge of heterogeneous environments. Mycologia. 1999;**9**:3-32. DOI: 10.2307/3761190

[63] Boddy L, Hiscox J. Fungal ecology: Principles and mechanisms of colonization and competition by saprotrophic fungi. Microbiology Spectrum. 2016;**4**(6):10-128. DOI: 10.1128/microbiolspec.funk-0019-2016

[64] Zabel RA, Morrell JJ. Wood Microbiology: Decay and its Prevention. San Diego: Academic Press; 1992. p. 476

[65] Lenhart K, Bunge M, Ratering S, Neu TR, Schüttmann I, Greule M, et al. Evidence for methane production by saprotrophic fungi. Nature Communications. 2012;**3**(1):1046. DOI: 10.1038/ncomms2049

[66] Juan-Ovejero R, Briones MJI, Öpik M. Fungal diversity in peatlands and its contribution to carbon cycling. Applied Soil Ecology. 2020;**146**:103393. DOI: 10.1016/j.apsoil.2019.103393

[67] Boldrini RF, Santos WO, Cruz ZM, Ramos AC. Bases da associação micorrízica orquidóide. Natureza Online. 2010;**8**(3):140-145

[68] Dantas BL, Weber OB, Neto JPM, Rossetti AG, Pagano MC. Diversidade de fungos micorrízicos arbusculares em pomar orgânico no semiárido cearense. Ciência Rural. 2015;**45**:1480-1486. DOI: 10.1590/0103-8478cr20130097

[69] Leonel LV et al. Biorremediação do solo. Revista Terra & Cultura: Cadernos de Ensino e Pesquisa. 2018;**26**(51):37-52

[70] Soares IA, Flores AC, Mendonça MM, Barcelos RP, Baroni S. Fungos na biorremediação de áreas degradadas. Arquivos do Instituto Biológico. 2020;**78**:341-350. DOI: 10.1590/1808-1657v78p3412011

[71] Lima DF, Oliveira OMC, Cruz Manoel JM. Utilização dos fungos na biorremediação de substratos contaminados por petróleo: estado da arte. Cadernos de Geociências. Salvador, BA, Brazil: Universidade Federal da Bahia (UFBA); 2011

[72] Carvalho AKF. Avaliação do potencial do fungo filamentoso *Mucor circinelloides* como fonte de lipase e lipídios para a produção de biodiesel dentro do conceito de biorrefinaria [Tese]. Brazil: Universidade de São Paulo; 2015

[73] Abreu JAS, Rodovida AFS, Pamphile JA. Fungos de interesse: aplicações biotecnológicas. Uningá Review. 2015;**21**(1):55-59

[74] Moizinho CV, Silva GA, Guimarães LL, Santos VG. O uso de microdosagem de psilocibina no tratamento de transtornos mentais. Unisanta BioScience. 2024;**13**(1):72-84

[75] Alves PH, Araújo JV, Guimarães MP, Assis RCL, Sarti P, Campos AK. Aplicação de formulação do fungo predador de nematoides *Monacrosporium thaumasium* (Drechsler, 1937) no controle de nematoides de bovinos. Arquivo Brasileiro de Medicina Veterinária e Zootecnia. 2003;**55**:568-573. DOI: 10.1590/S0102-09352003000500009

[76] Ferreira LV, Silva MA, Gurgel ESC, Santos JU, Brito EG, Mesquita MAP. Importância do Parque Estadual do Utinga Camilo Viana para a conservação das espécies de plantas e fungos da região metropolitana de Belém, Pará, Brasil. Boletim Do Museu Paraense Emílio Goeldi - Ciências Naturais. 2022;**17**(1):165-205. DOI: 10.46357/bcnaturais.v17i1.779

[77] Quezada ML, Lopez-Mayorga R, Sunum R, Perez-Silva E, Papa M, Herreira JP, et al. Macrofungos como indicadores da qualidade do habitat e a mudança climática. In: Jesus MA, Matsuura ABJ, Oliveira JGS, Gasparotto L, Lima-Neto RG, Rocha LC, editors. Conhecimento, Conservação e uso dos fungos, Manaus. Manaus, Amazonas, Brazil: Editora INPA; 2019. p. 97

[78] Moreno GS. Indicadores sociais, mudanças na paisagem e clima: efeitos em doenças emergentes e reemergentes [Tese]. Porto Seguro, BA: Universidade Federal do Sul da Bahia; 2022. Available from: https://repositorio.ifba.edu.br/jspui/handle/123456789/292

[79] Mendonza AYG, Silva VV, Lima RA, Lima JPS. Potencialidades Biotecnológicas dos Fungos da Amazônia Brasileira: Uma Revisão Sistemática. Diversitas Journal. 2022;7(4):2535-2551. DOI: 10.48017/dj.v7i4.2104

[80] Velho M. Fungos, processos e poéticas de interdependência. Revista ClimaCom. Desastres. Pesquisa-ensaios. 2023;**25**:1-21. Available from: https://climacom.mudancasclimaticas.net.br/fungos/

Section 2

Endophytic Fungi

Chapter 3

Endophytic Fungi: Taxonomy, Isolation, and Current Applications

Jorge Rojas López-Menchero, María Fé Andrés-Yeves, Azucena González-Coloma and Vicente González-García

Abstract

This chapter is a revision of the realm of endophytic fungi, focusing on how to approach the study of their biodiversity in relation to distribution, richness, host plant defense mechanisms, chemistry, and metabolomic profiles. We will revise the current isolation and identification methods available such as culture-dependent techniques and omics approaches including both targeted and functional metagenomics, and their comparison to give a holistic view of the endophytic fungal biome. Additionally, we will discuss their biotechnological potential for the production of bioactive natural products to be applied in plant protection (against nematodes, fungi, and insect control), soil restoration, or disease control practices based on microbial antagonists.

Keywords: fungal endophytes, omics, bioinformatics, natural products, plant protection

1. Introduction

An endophytic microorganism is commonly defined as a bacterium or fungus that spends most of its life cycle colonizing intra- or intercellularly the inner tissues of a given host plant, without causing apparent disease symptoms [1]. These organisms are present in all terrestrial plant species tested up to date and are considered ubiquitous and omnipresent throughout the whole plant kingdom. The diversity of this group of microorganisms can be remarkable; employing culture-dependent techniques, more than 100 endophytic fungal taxa per plant individual have been identified in some plant hosts, while this diversity can increase between 1 and 1.5 orders of magnitude when more resolution approaches related to the use of high-throughput sequencing methods are used in its characterization [2]. Another factor that influences the great diversity observed in endophytic fungal communities is geographical variation. It has been observed that species isolated from the same plant hosts tend to be different between different localities [3, 4]. The age of the plant host also has a certain effect on the composition of endophytic diversity. As the host lives longer, the exposure time to the fungal inoculum increases, accumulating a greater number of endophytic microorganisms in its tissues. It has been shown that the longest lived parts of a given plant species can harbor more endophytes than new tissues [5].

Another related concept with high biotechnological potential is the so-called chemical diversity that this type of fungal communities can harbor, as a consequence of their particular lifestyle and role played in the ecosystems in which they thrive [6]. This chemical diversity makes these species relatively unexplored sources of new natural products for application in medicine, agriculture, biotechnology, or industry [7]. Additionally, this endophytic fungal diversity has allowed in numerous studies the characterization and exploitation of microbial antagonists useful in conservation biological control programs within the framework of Integrated Pest Management approaches [8].

It is well known that some of the physiological and ecological roles played by endophytic fungal communities have to do with increasing the fitness or biological efficiency of the hosts they colonize, due to the production of certain functional metabolites. Like mycorrhizal species, endophytes interact with their hosts by promoting their growth, eliciting their response to certain environmental stresses (humidity, temperature, salinity, etc.), increasing their ability to resist attack by herbivores, or against infection by other pathogenic species of fungal origin [9]. In this sense, the ability of endophytic fungi to influence the interactions of host plants with their environment, as well as to modify their interaction processes with other pathogenic organisms, has been known for some time. In the last 10–20 years, numerous studies have shown that endophytic microorganisms can play a substantial role in the outcome of the different plant-pathogen interactions preceding the onset of the disease [10]. In this sense, various mechanisms have been described by which this type of fungi can prevent and/or limit the development of pathogens. For example, some endophytic species can induce systemic resistance and defense mechanisms against the attack of certain pathogens in their host plants [11], or even produce antibiotics capable of inhibiting the growth of other fungi [12]. Furthermore, endophytic species may eventually compete for space and nutrients with pathogen populations [13]. Finally, another key aspect of the biology of this type of organism is that some plant pathogens can behave as endophytes at some point in their life cycle [14]. This question is of great interest for the study of plant infection phenomena. Among all the fungal taxa that can penetrate and colonize the tissues of a given host, only a small proportion of them, the pathogens themselves, trigger pathogenesis.

The present work deals with different aspects of this large type of microorganism, from certain general aspects such as the definition and characteristics of this lifestyle, some milestones in the history of their research, or key aspects of its biology and distribution, going through a review of the different approaches and methodologies usually used in its sampling, isolation, and characterization, to finally review some of the main practical applications derived from its knowledge and exploitation, including human and animal medicine or industry, with special emphasis on sustainable approaches in agroecosystems (natural products, biological control agents, etc.).

2. Endophytic fungi: definition, main characteristics, infection mode

Fungi are widespread organisms with the ability of growing in multiple niches. Regarding their lifestyle, fungi can be divided in different groups: saprobes (growing on dead or dying material); pathogens (mainly infecting animals or plants); symbiotic (in beneficial interaction with other organisms); epiphytes (living on the surface of plants); or endophytes (inhabiting plants with no sign of harm or disease).

This chapter will provide an overview of key aspects regarding endophytic fungi. The main endophytic organisms are mostly bacteria and fungi, and in some cases, archaea and some protists [15]. Endophytic fungi are considered to be a polyphyletic group, but the genera and species encompassed in it can also be found among the aforementioned, including some that are traditionally considered pathogens or parasites. In addition to the classic definition of endophyte organisms, it is noteworthy to mention that in some cases, endophytic fungi may also be beneficial for the host plant. Thus, endophytic fungi can alter and increase the production of phytohormones, resulting in plant growth promotion and/or defense against pathogens. For instance, lettuce plants inoculated with an endophytic strain of *Penicillium pinophilum* aid in enhancing protection against *Verticillium*, resulting in a higher growth rate and reduced visible symptoms in leaves [16]. In another example, inoculation with two endophytes led wheat to induce systemic response and subsequent resistance to *Rhopalosiphum padi*, increasing the upregulation of defense-related genes and the content of jasmonic acid and other hormones and metabolites [17]. In some cases, during *in vitro* experiments, endophytic fungi do not show direct antagonistic effects against fungal phytopathogens, but their presence *in vivo* may prevent the infection from other fungi due to the occupancy of the same niches inside the plant [18, 19]. Since endophytes do not present any threat to plants, they are presented as a potential method in Integrated Pest Management (IPM) to develop more sustainable agricultural practices [20].

2.1 Transmission of endophytes

There are essentially two modes of transmission of fungal endophytes: vertical and horizontal. Vertical transmission refers to the transmission from the original plant to its descendance through the seed, while horizontal implies transmission either through soil, air or vectors, or through the pollen of another plant hosting this fungus [21]. In general, vertical transmission is less common, with most of the studied examples in the genus *Epichlöe* and its narrow relationship with tall fescue grasses [22, 23]. Nevertheless, this phenomenon is not exclusive to this genus, and it can be found in other endophytic fungi such as *Alternaria* and *Cladosporium*, among others [24, 25]. This transmission can be modulated by some factors that can be determinant for the process. Thus, plant genotype seems to play a major role, promoting the proliferation of certain taxa and/or communities on seeds and seedlings augmenting selective pressure for some species in favor of others [24]. Moreover, vertical transmission of endophytes seems to be important to reduce the presence of phytopathogenic fungi in seeds and plants. However, there are other secondary factors that can also modulate vertical transmission and settlement of fungal communities, such as host defense mechanisms [26], temperature [27] or water availability [28]. Regarding horizontal transmission, it is the most common way of endophyte dissemination into other plants. From an ecological point of view, horizontal transmission is very important to establish symbiotic relationships with other plants. While vertical transmission is only disseminating endophytic fungi through a genetic line, horizontal transmission can help their dispersion to wider areas or whole ecosystems, inside the same or different species [29]. Horizontal transmission might contribute to increased plant fitness and stress resistance in whole local populations such as forests or grasslands [30]. Apart from the natural ways of dispersion of fungi (soil, air, etc.), their dissemination is sometimes mediated by external vectors (i.e., insects), whose digestive tract can contain a diverse mycobiome that sometimes includes endophytic species that can pass to new plants during herbivory [31]. Some researchers hypothesize that the pollen microbiome may play a role in maintaining stable microbiomes within plants of the same species. Exploring its potential impact on the presence of plants across various ecosystems offers promising opportunities for future investigation in microbial ecology and how it can shape plant communities [32]. In any case, both strategies of transmission, vertical and horizontal, can frequently be found at the same time in the same fungal species, increasing its possibilities to disseminate through entire populations in an ecosystem [33].

2.2 Discovery and importance of endophytic fungi: *epichloe* and *Serendipita indica* as cases of study

Endophytes are very important for the development and fitness of the host plants. Thus, endophytic fungi may confer adaptability, protection, and enhanced nutrients intake to the plants they inhabit [34]. Probably, one of the first and most studied cases of fungal endophytes is the case of the genus *Epichlöe* (formerly *Neotyphodium).* One of the first hints of the beneficial relationship between endophyte and its host was documented in 1977 by Bacon et al. [35]. This studio was connecting the presence of *Epichlöe typhina* in tall fescue grasses with the diseases in cattle after consuming plants infected by this fungus. Subsequent studies determined that the toxicity was associated to the presence of multiple alkaloids inside of the plants, among other secondary metabolites, that had been produced by some fungi [36–38]. Later, some works determined that grasses infected with these fungi were predominant in pasture and outcompeted non-infected plants [39]. Additionally, some studies have connected the higher resistance of some plants to pests and diseases to their infection with *Epichlöe* and its secondary metabolites. For instance, one of the main compounds derived from this interaction, N-formoline, is toxic to insects. For example, decreased *in vitro* survival rate of *Stenotus rubrovittatus* in the presence of this compound [40], or the decreased survival of *Trigonotylus caelestialium* when this compound is present in plants, even at low doses [41]. A wide range of metabolites produced by these fungi can protect the plant against insect pests [42]. Apart from insects, *Epichlöe* has also been reported to reduce significantly the presence of other pathogens. For example, strong nematicidal effects have been observed against *Pratylenchus scribneri,* inducing a significant decrease in nematode population when the fungus was inhabiting the plant [43]. Similarly, other authors noted a decrease in *Meloidogyne javanica* infection in plants colonized by this fungus [44]. Furthermore, several authors have reported toxicity in some metabolites derived from *Epichlöe* against fungal phytopathogens such as *Phytophthora infestans* [45–47]. It has also been observed that some fungi that colonize plants are able to influence the bacterial microbiome of the soil where they develop [48, 49], being a potentially useful tool to reduce pathogenic microorganisms from the soil.

The root endophyte *Serendipita indica* (formerly *Piriformospora indica)* has been extensively proven to confer tolerance to biotic and abiotic stresses to its host plants. *Serendipita indica* can affect the pattern of production of phytohormones and plant secondary metabolites [50] which trigger and increase the plant response to biotic and abiotic stresses. For example, the colonization by this fungus improves *Arabidopsis thaliana* growth under salt stress, through the modulation of the expression levels of the main Na + and K+ ion channels [51]. Other study describes and characterizes two ENA ATPases proteins in *S. indica* involved in the molecular mechanism of tolerance against high salinity [52]. On the other hand, the inoculation of *Pinus taeda* plants with this fungi enhanced its tolerance to drought, changing the metabolome and proteome of the plant and increasing the protein content of the leaves and of several metabolites such as suberine and 2-oxocarboxylic acid among other flavonoids and organic acids that protect the plant from drought stress [53]. Besides this, *S. indica* colonization has been reported to increase nutrient uptake. Thus, in tobacco, it has been demonstrated that *S. indica* can enhance nitrogen uptake by inducing the expression of ammonium and nitrate transporter genes, promoting plant growth [54]. Similarly, the fungal colonization increases phosphorus intake, due to the transport to the host plant mediated by high affinity phosphate transporters [55], magnesium [56], zinc [57], or iron [58]. Conversely, *S. indica* reduces the accumulation of boron [59] and arsenic [60, 61] among other heavy metals that can be harmful to both plants and humans. In addition to the ability of inducing tolerance in host plants against biotic and abiotic stress, *S. indica* has also been proven as a potential tool for the biocontrol of insect pests. Thus, its presence in onion plants significantly reduced (>50%) the damage caused by *Spodoptera exigua*, promoting the defensive response through the upregulation of genes and routes related to defense and oxidative stress [62]. In the same way, *S. indica* enhanced herbivory resistance to *Cnaphalocrocis medinalis* through higher production of jasmonic acid and mitigation of oxidative stresses [63]. Furthermore, *S. indica* has been successfully applied in the biocontrol of other plant pests and pathogens such as root-knot nematodes or fungi. For example, root colonization by this fungus promotes cucumber tolerance to *Meloidogyne javanica* by modulating photosynthesis and salicylic hormone levels [64]. Several examples can also be found for biocontrol of fungi, for example, against some common pathogens such as *Verticillium dahliae* or *Fusarium graminearum* [65, 66].

In addition to the aforementioned examples, many other can be found in literature about endophytic fungi that are also known to improve the fitness and tolerance of the host plants to biotic and abiotic stresses: osmotic pressure due to salinity [67]; to heavy metals [68–70]; to drought [71–74]; to temperatures [74, 75]; to nutrient deficiency [76, 77] and to pests and pathogens [16, 17, 78].

2.3 Diversity of endophytic fungi

Based on the ratio of endophytes found in vascular plants, approximately up to 1 million fungal species are estimated to exist [79] but other authors set this number in up to 12 million [80]. Moreover, with the development of NGS methods (discussed later in this review), particularly shotgun metagenomics, numerous new species are being described as endophytes every year, making predictions far from accurate at this moment. Notwithstanding, the study of diversity of endophytic fungi can be challenging, especially due to the difficulty to determine if some species are real endophytes or latent pathogens. Additionally, classifying endophytes can be complex, requiring a multifaceted approach to their biology [79]. Latent pathogens are fungi that may become pathogenic at certain stages of a plant's development but remain harmless for most of the time. Often, additional pathogenicity assays are required to determine whether an isolated fungus is endophytic or pathogenic [81, 82].

Some of the most extended fungal pathogenic species along most ecosystems have an equivalent endophytic strain that is only not harming the plants they inhabit, but their presence is favorable to their host. Several cases of this phenomenon can be found in literature. For instance, *Fusarium* species infect up to 120 horticultural plants [83], causing wilt disease and head blight disease, among others. It is a soilborne fungus spread in multiple agrosystems worldwide and its infection and mycotoxins cause important crop and economic losses [84–86]. There have been described several strains of *Fusarium spp.* with beneficial effects on its host: *Fusarium sp.* isolates from *Withania somnifera* were reported to display growth promotion effects on tomatoes in addition to disease suppression ability against other pathogenic *Fusarium* strains [87]. *Fusarium* is also one of the main pathogens in bananas, but when the effects of the application of non-pathogenic *F. oxysporum* strains were studied, banana crop yields were enhanced along with a reduction in the populations of phytopathogenic nematodes in soil and their damage on the plants [88]. Another example of fungi considered a pathogen displaying endophytic behavior is *Verticillium.* Species of this genus also cause important economic losses in agriculture every year [89]. The strain Vt305 of *V. isaacii* demonstrated to be effective in controlling wilt disease caused by *V. longisporum*, reducing severe disease symptoms in both greenhouse and field conditions [90]. Differences in endophytic/pathogenic behavior of *V. dahliae* have been studied, finding that this species can be found as an endophyte or a pathogen depending on its host, suggesting a possible process of speciation based on endophytic specialization from pathogenic lines [91]. Additionally, several other examples of traditional pathogens with endophytic behaviors have been documented for several fungi genus such as *Alternaria* [92], *Colletotrichum* [76, 93], and *Acremonium* [94, 95], among many others.

Most endophytic fungi are considered generalists, capable of inhabiting a wide range of host plants, whereas there are relatively fewer fungi that are specialized to specific host plant species. Certain species and genera of fungi frequently appear and commonly form an important part of the host plant's microbiome. This includes fungal genera such as *Fusarium*, *Trichoderma*, and *Aspergillus*, among others reported in the literature. In broad terms, abundance and diversity of fungi can be studied in several scales. Globally, many environmental factors shape endophytic communities in different hosts and ecosystems [96]. Essentially, the highest diversity and abundance of fungal endophytes can be found in tropical areas (being considered as hyper diverse group), while in colder areas, its diversity and abundance decrease [97]. Furthermore, there is a higher tendency to find greater host-endophyte specificity in Arctic and boreal zones than in tropical and temperate zones [98]. This suggests that generalist endophytic fungi are more likely to be more abundant in warm and temperate zones, while the relative abundance of specialist endophytic fungi tends to increase in colder ones. Furthermore, it is noteworthy that islands and endemic plants may serve as very potential reservoirs of yet undiscovered endophytic fungi with prospective applications [99–101].

When reducing the scale of the study to the host plant, differences can also be observed. Thus, in the different parts of the plants, there are differences in the communities of fungal endophytes. Generally, several authors have observed higher abundance and diversity of fungi species in roots than in aerial parts [102–104]. This is likely attributable to soil being a primary entry point for endophytic fungi into plants, as well as the presence of various fungi that can function both as saprobes in the soil and as endophytes [105]. As a matter of fact, there frequently exists partial overlapping between soil and endophytic fungi communities [106]. However, sometimes, diversity and abundance patterns in host plants are occasionally affected by external factors, that is, infection by pathogens [107].

2.4 Insights in the interaction between endophyte and its host

The interaction between endophytes and plants is not merely the result of a random arrival of the fungus near the plant. Rather, in many cases, it is an interaction driven by bidirectional communication between fungi and plants, often resulting from mutual signaling mechanisms. Given the ability of plants to detect microbe-associated molecular patterns (MAMPs), this interaction can sometimes be promoted by the plant itself for its benefit. For instance, the production of root exudates rich in chemoattractants eases the entrance of endophytes to the plants [108]. In some other cases, to colonize a plant, endophytic fungi alter host metabolism, by decreasing the defensive response or shaping the host metabolism [109–112]. For instance, colonization by some endophytes can modulate gene expression in plants, finding downregulation of some biotic stress and primary metabolism genes [113]. Besides, the production of certain small secreted proteins or SSPs by endophytic fungi seems important to reduce the defensive mechanism of the plants and facilitate host colonization, [114–116]. In fact, in some cases, SSP expression may be found to be higher in endophytic fungi than in pathogenic strains. Additionally, hormone production patterns can also be altered by the entrance of determined endophytic fungi in plants [117]. Plant hormones seem to have a key role in this interaction, particularly abscisic acid (ABA), jasmonic acid (JA), and salicylic acid (SA). Hu and Bidochka [118] reported ABA as an hormone capable of modulating different plant defensive responses during colonization either endophytes or pathogens. When an endophytic fungus colonized the plant, ABA-related genes were downregulated, while when a pathogenic one did, they were upregulated. Furthermore, in their study, the external application of ABA was used to hypothesize its potential as a useful tool for promoting positive endophyte colonization, demonstrating that ABA treatment decreased endophytic colonization while increasing pathogen colonization when applied to the plants. Similar effects have been demonstrated for SA, where its exogenous application suppressed *Epichlöe* in leaves of ryegrass [109]. In this context, it has been demonstrated that *Epichlöe* is able to suppress the SA pathway and simultaneously increase auxin production. This highlights its ability to manipulate plant hormone pathways and suggests that the ability to shape and suppress plant defense responses is essential for successful endophytic colonization [119]. Additionally, it underscores the importance of defense suppression in the evolution of endophytic fungi and plants, as SA application also reduced the presence of characteristic *Epichlöe* alkaloids in leaves, leading to lower pest resistance.

In addition to alterations in primary plant metabolism during the interaction, Horizontal Gene Transfer (HGT) between fungi and plants is a phenomenon yet to be elucidated. In the past, some authors proposed HGT as a hypothesis to explain why some endophytic fungi were able to produce compounds of their hosts. Several authors have reported the importance of HGT in the evolution of certain organisms. For instance, non-pathogenic strains of *Fusarium* may become pathogenic due to the transfer of chromosomes from pathogenic strains when cultured together [120], and conversely, loss of accessory chromosomes may lead pathogenic fungi to become endophytes [121]. HGT has been observed between bacteria-bacteria [122], fungus-fungus [123], and bacteria-fungus [124], but it is a very rare phenomenon between fungi and plants.

Additionally, in the last years, it has come to attention how mycoviruses could be modifying the genome and behavior of endophytic fungi. The mycovirus (PtCV1) from an endophytic strain of the fungus *Pestalotiopsis theae* conferred high resistance to the host plants against the virulent pathogen *P. theae* strains and reduced the virulence of its fungal host [125]. Similarly, plants colonized by a hypovirulent *Sclerotinia sclerotiorum* strain, with mycovirus (SlaGemV-1), showed a resistant phenotype to virulent *S. sclerotiorum* infection [126]. Therefore, plant immunity induced by endophytic colonization of mycovirus-induced hypovirulent fungal pathogen provides an alternative approach to biological control of plant diseases caused by fungi.

The role of HGT in inter-kingdom interactions remains an area of significant interest and debate, especially due to the absence of knowledge about how some fungi are able to produce compounds of the plants they inhabit. The case of taxol is likely one of the best-known instances of endophytic fungi producing a plant molecule. In 1993, Stierle et al. described the ability of *Taxomyces andreanae*, a fungus isolated from *Taxus brevifolia*, of producing taxol, an important drug used in cancer therapy [127]. There are reports of other taxol-producing fungi, and some authors have hypothesized that HGT could explain this phenomenon [128]. Nevertheless, current evidence does not fully support this hypothesis, as the fungal and plant taxol pathways appear to be a case of convergent evolution [129]. However, there are other cases of HGT between endophytic fungi and plants, such as a ß-1,6-glucanase (an enzyme that degrades fungal cell walls) [130] or the Fusarium Head Blight resistance gene [131]. Additionally, apart from taxol, other plant compounds have been observed to be produced by endophytic fungi [132, 133]. These observations are consistent with the hypothesis and keep it viable for further studies.

3. Isolation and identification of endophytic fungi

In the last five decades, the term endophyte, or more specifically endophytic fungi and many of the variants associated with the concept (endophytic colonization, endosphere, endophytism, etc.) have become more familiar and present in scientific and popular literature, to refer in a precise way to these fungal microbial communities (also for bacterial ones) that, as another type of symbiosis defined as the "coexistence of different organisms," names the lifestyle of those fungi that live asymptomatically in the internal tissues of higher plants. Regarding the different isolation techniques of this type of endophytic microbial diversity, the different methods commonly employed have generally pivoted until now on aspects related to the way of sampling, treating, and surface sterilizing the plant materials of origin, or on the composition and selectivity of synthetic nutritional media used in the management (isolation, sporulation, maintenance, etc.) of these microorganisms. On the other hand, as for other groups of fungi, the identification of different taxonomic entities has long been a laborious task that requires deep multidisciplinary knowledge (anatomy, cytology, histology, nomenclature, etc.), which usually limited speed and resolution of reliable taxonomic determinations. The arrival and generalization toward the end of the 90s of molecular characterization techniques greatly improved the speed of taxonomic determination work, while the phylogenetic affinities existing between the groups of organisms studied were drawn more precisely. More recently, it has been shown that the sequence diversity existing in small DNA fragments of standardized genomic regions allows diagnostic identification in numerous groups of microorganisms (including both eukaryotes and prokaryotes) [134], which today we know it as DNA Barcoding. This approach, based on a standardization of identification systems using these genetic barcodes, has led to greater confidence in the diagnosis and identity of species, facilitating numerous practical applications, including the study of fungal endophyte populations. Finally, the generalization of the use of high-throughput sequencing techniques, based largely on the identification of organisms from the mentioned barcode sequences, has also allowed, in the case of endophytic fungi, mass characterization, and identification of microbial diversity in a much more efficient way than that obtained through classic culture-dependent microbiological techniques.

3.1 Isolating methods of endophytic fungi. Classical taxonomic characterization and molecular systematics approaches

3.1.1 Isolation and culture

As a rule, it has been widely accepted up to date that some basic microbiological procedures are essential to yield the greatest amount of microbial diversity possible when studying endophytic communities in each plant species. Most of these methods are routine protocols in a microbiology context, not especially difficult for well-trained personnel [106]. The first critical step in the isolation procedures has to do with the processing of fresh plant material in good condition, where there must be an acceptable balance between the degree of desiccation and aeration of the samples, to avoid both the death of the tissue and its colonization by contaminant microorganisms. Following these handling protocols, removing epiphytic, contaminating fungal species usually present in plant tissues must be carried out by surface sterilization methods to ensure the isolation of true endophytic diversity. The most employed methods for surface sterilization of plant tissues are based on the sequential immersion of materials in EtOH and NaOCl solutions. Other chemical agents less employed for removing epiphytic microorganisms are mercury chloride ($HgCl_2$), hydrogen peroxide (H_2O_2), paraquat, or 1% peroxyacetic acid (CH_3COOOH) in 30% ethanol [2]. Some authors have proposed alternative protocols for surface sterilization that include alternative germicidal agents such as the sequential use of calcium hypochlorite, sodium hydrogen carbonate, and finally sodium azide [135]. Together with the dip in the mentioned germicidal agents, the processing can be completed with washing materials with sterile distilled water either before or after treatment with sterilizing solutions. In the case of very delicate plant tissues or for those that do not withstand the action of ethanol or bleach well, cleaning with serial washings only with sterile deionized water or the continuous action of running tap water is usually indicated [106]. In these latter cases, it is usually necessary to use a synthetic isolation medium supplemented with some type of antibiotic. Another reported alternative method for removing surface contaminants consists of intense washing and subsequent sonication of the tissues before plating and incubation [136]. The immersion times and concentrations of sterilizing solutions of ethanol and bleach will be a combination of each plant studied (monocots, dicots, lichens, mosses, ferns, etc.) and the type and nature of the tissue or organ processed (leaves, stems, twigs, trunk, roots, leaf litter, etc.). In the literature, there are numerous examples of surface sterilization protocols for endophytic fungi (dipping times, concentrations, etc.) as a guide [106].

Following the surface sterilization processes, the design and choice of incubation, culture, and isolation protocols for endophytic microorganisms are key when it comes to characterizing the greatest amount of fungal microbial diversity possible. In this sense, the size of the plant sample under study is crucial, since a clear and direct relationship is established between it and the recovery/identification rate of species. In fact, it is commonly assumed that the smaller the sample size, the greater the isolated cultivable diversity, while on the contrary, the larger the size of the material analyzed, the possibility of overlooking rare or very slow-growing species will be greater [106].

As a rule, fragments of variable size of host tissues are usually placed on the surface of certain synthetic nutritive agar medium in a way that ensures a distance between fragments that allows the emergence and growth of individual fungal colonies. To avoid overlap and cross-contamination in colonies due to the existence of fast-growing species, the use of microwell plates is highly recommended, in combination with a maximum fragmentation of plant material. These processes of cutting and separating tissues into the smallest possible fragments are often laborious and time-consuming in the laboratory, so alternative material atomization methods can be used. One of the most frequently used is the maceration of the tissues, the filtration of particles, and their subsequent dilution and plating. This is a technique originally developed for high-throughput bacterial cultivation of slow-growing bacteria that has been adapted by several authors [137–139], to improve the recovery rates of culturable fungi from certain complex substrata.

Concerning culture media employed to isolate, maintain, and characterize endophytic fungi, synthetic routinary microbiology media are considered to be suitable for a primary recovery and isolation of fungal endophytes, also for subsequent subculturing and purify isolated strains. In this sense, PDA is the most used and widespread medium for these purposes [2], although another commonly used media is Malt Extract Agar (1–2%), sometimes in combination with yeast extract [106]. Other less common synthetic culture media used for the isolation of this type of microorganisms would be Agar containing Murashige and Skoog (MS) vitamins and sucrose [140], Hagem Minimal Medium [141], Czapek medium [142], Tryptone Soybean Agar, Tryptone Bovine Extract Agar, and Luria-Bertani (also known as LB broth) medium [143]. In addition to its composition of basic nutrients and depending on the type of endophytic diversity to be studied, the use of certain supplements in isolation media is also a common practice. Thus, the employment of microbial growth inhibitors such as fungistatics or antibiotics, is usually common practice in the primary isolation of strains. The former are usually used to delay the emergence of fast growing fungal species that can often hide and prevent the isolation of slower-growing taxa, and substances such as Dichloran, Pimaricin, Benomyl, certain antibiotics such as Cyclosporin A or Amphotericin are usually used. Other compounds include surfactants (i.e., benzyltrimethylammonium hydroxide, sodium dodecyl sulfate) and organic acids (tannic acid, lactic acid) to be employed as differentially selective agents in culture media [106]. Regarding the control of bacterial growth, it is usually common practice to supplement the isolation media with one or several broad-spectrum antibiotics such as sodium benzylpenicillin, chloramphenicol, streptomycin, gentamicin, or tetracycline [2].

After purification and obtaining in pure culture of the different isolates, these are usually classified in a first stage based on their micro- and macromorphological diagnostic characteristics in culture, as the basis of a classic taxonomic approach. Thus, endophytic fungi are usually identified at the species level using firstly morphological characterization combined with subsequent molecular methods. Vegetative morphological characters in plate culture usually include pigmentation (including the colony reverse), odor, topology (texture, margin, type, and growth rate), or the cardinal temperatures of the colonies in different axenic media [2], together with the description (when they are available) of the different reproductive (sexual and asexual) or resistance (sclerotia, chlamydospores, etc.) structures [144]. However, for many of the endophytic species routinely isolated, the aforementioned reproductive structures could not be available and the different isolates usually present as sterile mycelia, which can be subjected to certain techniques to promote their sporulation, from the use of specific culture media (including plant components or hydrophobic elements, etc.) [145, 146] to the exposure to certain lengths of UV light [147].

3.1.2 Taxonomic identification of fungal endophytes

Even when an acceptable number of diagnostic macro- and micromorphological characters are available for classical taxonomic identification, this can present different problems, since classical taxonomic work not performed by specialists in fungal systematics can be effective in establishing identifications at the genus or family, but often presents problems in classifying lower taxonomic levels (specific or infra-specific), especially in complex and/or highly diverse groups, where morphological characters can be misleading or insufficiently diagnostic due to the existence of phenomena such as hybridization, cryptic speciation, or evolutionary convergence [148]. As a consequence, it is necessary to have more precise methods for the identification of fungal isolates based on molecular techniques [149].

Although, in the past, molecular techniques have been applied to connect anamorph and teleomorph phases in endophytic species such as Random Amplification of Polymorphic DNA (RAPD) [150], currently, the selective amplification of the ribosomal ITS region and other useful genomic areas and the subsequent analysis and comparison of these sequences, has become the most widespread method of taxonomic identification of isolates, due to its universality, reproducibility, and ease of automating processes. Basically, the routine work of molecular characterization of endophytic isolates involves a series of generic processes and sequential steps, ranging from the extraction of the genomic DNA of the microorganisms to be identified (normally from pure cultures or to a lesser extent from complex environmental samples), the subsequent selective amplification using universal or specific primers by PCR (conventional, RT-PCR, etc.) of certain genomic regions (conserved or not), the sequencing of the PCR products, their subsequent processing and comparison with public databases (preferably curated and taxonomically supervised), and to finally determine and infer both the taxonomic identity and the phylogenetic relationships existing between the characterized species [2]. Although not without limitations (especially present in certain groups of filamentous Ascomycetes and to a lesser extent Basidiomycetes) [151, 152], the ribosomal ITS region that includes its three most commonly employed components, the LSU (26-28S) and SSU (18S) fragments and the ITS region (including the internal spacers ITS1 and 2 and the 5.8S region), is currently considered the most preferred molecular DNA marker to identify fungi, being accepted as a primary barcode region for mass and routinary identification. These DNA barcodes (massively used in other groups of living organisms) are short (400–600 bp), universal, and standardized DNA sequences that are easily amplifiable (unlike other more conserved genomic regions), with a common presence in different groups of the Kingdom Fungi and related organisms, but highly divergent at the species level [153]. For the identification of certain groups and genera that are especially complex or that contain numerous cryptic species (e.g., *Fusarium*, *Cladosporium*, *Penicillium*, *Rhizoctonia*, *Verticillium*), in addition to the use of these DNA barcodes based on the ribosomal ITS region, the sequencing of fragments from other protein-coding genomic regions (i.e., tef-1, RPB1, RPB2, CaM, tub1/BenA) is necessary to, through a multiloci phylogenetic analysis, clarify the molecular systematics of highly complex groups [154].

3.2 New methods of analysis of endophytic mycobiota: amplicon and shotgun metagenomics. Present application of bioinformatics and potential in the future. Transcriptomic analysis of the plant in the presence/absence of certain endophytes

Among the new techniques for analysis and description of endophytic microbial communities, next-generation sequencing (NGS) methods currently play a crucial role, providing experimental evidence on their diversity, population structure, abundance, metabolic functionality, or ecological role played in the ecosystems they inhabit [155]. Using this type of approach and employing DNA from complex environmental samples (soil, plant tissues, water, etc.), complete microgenomes can be sequenced simultaneously and relatively fast [156]. In purely taxonomic metagenomics (metabarcoding), sequences produced from amplicons of genomic regions of universal DNA barcodes are assigned to Operational Taxonomic Units (OTUs) according to a nucleotide similarity threshold by comparison with curated taxonomic databases [157]. Along with these types of approaches, Shotgun metagenomics allows sequencing the entire genomes of the whole microbial population from a total genomic DNA sample, allowing the identification and annotation of all microbial genes, providing additional information on the potential functionality of each microbiome studied, including the different metabolic pathways present in the microbiome of a given environmental sample [158].

These metagenomic approaches have revolutionized the analysis of endophytic communities without the use of laboratory microbiological routines, providing a more complete view of the microbial composition of plants [159]. In the specific case of Shotgun metagenomics, the simultaneous sequencing of complete genomes has allowed us to begin to access knowledge of the so-called deep biodiversity of microorganisms, made up of all those taxa (and their associated genes) that are usually discarded in metagenomic analyses by not having homologies in the available sequence databases. All this taxonomic and functional diversity probably represents most of the existing microbial diversity [160]. The first studies on endophyte metagenomics date back to 2013, although the generalization and progressive accessibility of NGS methods have rapidly stimulated the taxonomic, functional, and ecological characterization of endophytic (fungal and bacterial) metagenomes. In the last 5–10 years, analyses of microbial communities associated with all types of environments have multiplied, including the inner compartments of different organs and plant tissues [156]. Furthermore, the progressive preference in this type of study for the use of shotgun metagenomics is allowing us to highlight and exploit the potential of the metabolism of this type of microorganisms, in aspects such as knowledge of their secondary metabolism, their biochemical diversity or evolutionary significance [161].

Regarding the development and application of bioinformatics solutions and their potential for the analysis of metagenomic data for the study of endophytic communities, the need to process and manage large datasets has led to the development of computational tools and pipelines capable to integrate into single platforms (QUIIME, Galaxy, etc.), tasks such as the processing of raw sequences, the analysis and taxonomic assignment of marker genes, the evaluation and statistical analysis of diversity, or the prediction of ecological roles and aptitudes of the different OTUs. In the case of Shotgun metagenomics, data analysis is usually more complex than studies based on amplicons, since there are usually numerous difficulties in the assembly and annotation of metagenomes obtained *de novo*, where only a small percentage of the coding genes can be accurately identified. To overcome these obstacles, there are currently different bioinformatics tools such as assemblers (SOAP, Ray Meta, Meta Velvet, Meta SPAdes, etc.), programs for grouping sequence fragments (Kraken, MaxBin2, Meta Bat, etc.), or tools for classification and annotation of metagenomes (PRODIGAL, MetaGenMark, SEED, KEGG, COG, etc.) [162].

In addition to culture-independent genomic approaches, other disciplines such as Transcriptomics or Metabolomics are currently being used to obtain a more complete view of the functioning and ecological role of endophytic microbial communities. This type of methodologies allows us to analyze the levels of gene expression both in an entire community and only for certain specific species of microorganisms, or to characterize the biochemical profiles of a given community, revealing its metabolic state in a certain time frame [163]. In this way, transcriptomics can inform us of alterations in gene expression related to the establishment of fungal-plant mutualism relationships [164], pathogenesis phenomena [165], elicitation of the defensive response in plants [166, 167], or adaptability to different abiotic stresses [168, 169]. Interestingly, all these phenomena can be better understood and explained today with comparative gene expression analyses, either at the level of the plant transcriptome in the presence/absence of certain microorganisms or in the case of the fungal transcriptome in interaction or outside of the plant host studied [170].

4. Uses of endophytic fungi

Endophytic fungi possess numerous biosynthetic gene clusters that possess genes encoding various enzymes, transcription factors, etc., in their genome, responsible for the production of secondary metabolites. The discovery of the anticancer product taxol was a landmark in endophyte research and established potential of the metabolism of plant-associated endophytes. Plant-associated endophytes are recognized reservoirs of plant-derived natural products and novel metabolites of pharmacological and agricultural significance. Endophytic fungi-mediated biosynthesis of well-known metabolites includes taxol from *Taxomyces andreanae*, azadirachtin A and B from *Eupenicillium parvum*, vincristine from *Fusarium oxysporum*, quinine from *Phomopsis sp*. [171, 172], and ginsenosides [173]. Furthermore, synthetic biology engineering of endophytes for yield enhancement has been proposed as a prospective area of research to improve the yield of valuable compounds [174].

Antimicrobial compounds: Compounds with activity against microorganisms have been isolated from both endophytic fungi and actinomycetes. Specifically, the presence of bioactive metabolites with unique skeletons in endophytic fungi could contribute to the prevention of antimicrobial resistance. The major classes of metabolites reported include anthraquinone, sesquiterpenoid, chromone, xanthone, phenols, quinones, quinolone, piperazine, coumarins, and cyclic peptides [175–177]. However, only a limited number of these compounds have been subjected to comprehensive studies regarding their mechanisms of action against bacterial cells, their effects on antibiotic-resistant bacteria, and the identification of biosynthetic gene clusters responsible for synthesizing these secondary metabolites [178].

Anticancer: There is a high diversity of plant-associated endophytic fungi in nature that are potent producers of anticancer compounds, including terpenoids, flavonoids, alkaloids, phenolic compounds, quinines, steroids, with relevance in chemoprevention and as modulators of miRNA [179]. Some of these anticancer compounds, such as paclitaxel, camptothecin, vinblastine, vincristine, podophyllotoxin, and their derivatives, are currently being used clinically. By increasing the yield of specific compounds with genetic engineering and other biotechnologies, endophytic fungi could be a promising, prolific source of anticancer drugs [180].

Additional medicinal effects: Antiviral fungal endophyte secondary metabolites have potential as inhibitors of various HIV-1 target sites [181]. Some studies describe the presence of extracts and metabolites against diabetes mellitus in fungal endophytes [182], antileishmanial, and antitrypanosomal [183].

Plant protection and biocontrol: Endophytes can directly stimulate plant growth by producing phytohormones or stimulate plant growth by increasing the availability of soil nutrients to plants. Endophytes may also help suppress diseases in plants directly by neutralizing environmental toxic elements, and by inhibiting plant pathogens by antagonistic action, or indirectly by stimulating induced plant systemic resistance. Beneficial fungal endophytes improve plant performance, a condition that seems to be magnified in the presence of stress. There is a clear potential for symbiotically modifying crop plants as a strategy to develop more tolerant varieties to face stress and eventually increase the quality of agricultural products [184]. Fungal endophytes used as bioinoculants (bioformulations of selected microbial strains) confer various benefits to the host, such as elicitation of the immune response, mineralization of essential nutrients, and promotion of plant growth. To design bioformulations, genomics, transcriptomics, metabolomics, proteomics, and microbiome modulation strategies (gene editing and metabolic reconstruction) can be used in synthesizing microbial consortia by evaluating the role of structural and functional elements of communities in a controlled manner [185, 186].

Natural compounds produced by endophytes as secondary metabolites are beneficial to their hosts and can be externally produced for plant protection as an indirect effect [187]. Among the potential applications of fungal endophyte, secondary metabolites are antifungal and insecticidal, among others [188–190].

Enzymatic activity and biotransformation: Endophytic fungi exhibit notable enzymatic activity and biotransformation capabilities. Beyond producing a wide range of secondary metabolites applicable in agriculture and medicine through submerged fermentation in culture media, they can also produce compounds of interest by transforming waste and by-products into compounds of interest such as polyphenols and terpenoids, among others [191]. For instance, an endophytic strain of *Penicillium rubens* can produce genistein, a versatile compound with various applications, from the wastes of *Cajanus cajan* [192]. Similarly, through fermentation of orange-peel residues with *Alternaria arborescens,* transaminase enzymes with economic interest have been produced. It is noteworthy to mention the use of endophytic fungi in saponins production (10.2174/0113892010247700230919053439; [193–195]). Other endophytic enzymes with potential use in the industry have been described in the literature [196–198].

Additionally, their flexible enzymatic activity makes them a valuable asset in bioremediation. Free and inoculated endophytic fungi have been used in the bioremediation of cyanotoxins [199], polycyclic aromatic hydrocarbons [200], endocrine disruptive compounds [201], and lead and cadmium contamination [202, 203], among others.

Notably, a recent study explored the utilization of an endophytic fungus in winemaking as a carrier, reporting enhancements in aroma, polyphenols, and antioxidant capacity [204]. These findings provide significant insights for investigating the application of endophytic fungi and their enzymes in food technology.

5. Conclusions

Endophytic fungi constitute a group of microorganisms associated with practically all terrestrial plant species, whose importance and specific weight in the structure and ecosystems (including agroecosystems) have been being unraveled in the last 50–60 years. Some of the first species described and studied as endophytes have served as study models to further understand plant-microorganism relationships, allowing a more exact understanding of the processes that trigger pathogenic or mutualistic behavior. Currently, we know more precisely aspects such as the existing enormous diversity of this group of fungi, their distribution in the different plant tissues and compartments, what their seasonal patterns are, or how the composition and structure of endophytic populations change and evolve as their host plants do. The routine incorporation of molecular methods in fungal systematics has allowed the implementation of relatively simple and rapid protocols for the taxonomic identification of isolates, standardizing and universalizing approaches such as the determination of species based on the use of DNA barcodes. In a subsequent step, the generalization in the recent years of the use of high-throughput sequencing techniques has allowed, in addition to reveal and identify an amount of microbial diversity that is difficult to characterize employing only culture-dependent methods, to study the functionality of this type of fungal communities. In this sense, the incorporation of this and other omics into the studies of endophytic fungi allows us to discover new bioactive substances and compounds of interest and potential produced by these microorganisms (and their applications in agriculture, drug discovery, bioremediation, etc.), or unravel the complex interactions between microorganisms and the plants that host them, increasing our knowledge about the molecular bases of these relationships. These methods also allow us to elucidate the key role of the microbiome in the ecological adaptability and fitness of its plant hosts (to defend itself against biotic or abiotic stresses), to introduce the paradigm of "holobiont" understood as a biological unit composed of the sum of both the plant and its microbial genomes, or the role of microorganisms in providing ecosystemic services in the ecosystems they inhabit.

Acknowledgements

Jorge Rojas López-Menchero has been supported by a predoctoral contract FPI associated with the project PID2019-106222RB-C31 funded by MCIN/AEI/10.13039/501100011033 and FSE "El FSE invierte en tu futuro."

Author details

Jorge Rojas López-Menchero[1,2], María Fé Andrés-Yeves[1], Azucena González-Coloma[1] and Vicente González-García[3*]

1 Instituto de Ciencias Agrarias, CSIC, Madrid, Spain

2 Escuela Técnica Superior de Ingeniería Agronómica, Alimentaria y de Biosistemas, Universidad Politécnica de Madrid, Avda. Puerta de Hierro, Madrid, Spain

3 Centro de Investigación y Tecnología Agroalimentaria de Aragón (CITA), Instituto Agroalimentario de Aragón—IA2 (CITA-Universidad de Zaragoza), Zaragoza, Spain

*Address all correspondence to: vgonzalezg@cita-aragon.es

References

[1] Zabalgogeazcoa I. Fungal endophytes and their interaction with plant pathogens: A review. Spanish Journal of Agricultural Research. 2008;**6**:138-146

[2] dos Reis JBA, Lorenzi AS, do Vale HMM. Methods used for the study of endophytic fungi: A review on methodologies and challenges, and associated tips. Archives of Microbiology. 2022;**204**(11):675

[3] Collado J, Platas G, González I, Peláez F. Geographical and seasonal influences on the distribution of fungal endophytes in *Quercus ilex*. New Phytologist. 1999;**144**(3):525-532. Available from: https://www.onlinelibrary.wiley.com/doi/full/10.1046/j.1469-8137.1999.00533.x

[4] Collado J, Platas G, Peláez F. Host specificity in fungal endophytic populations of *Quercus ilex* and *Quercus faginea* from Central Spain. Nova Hedwigia. 2000;**71**(3-4):421-430

[5] Arnold AE, Mejía LC, Kyllo D, Rojas EI, Maynard Z, Robbins N, et al. Fungal endophytes limit pathogen damage in a tropical tree. National Academy of Sciences of the United States of America. 2003;**100**(26):15649-15654

[6] Tan RX, Zou WX. Endophytes: A rich source of functional metabolites (1987 to 2000). Natural Product Reports. 2001;**18**(4):448-459

[7] Strobel G, Daisy B. Bioprospecting for microbial endophytes and their natural products. Microbiology and Molecular Biology Reviews. 2003;**67**(4):491-502

[8] Backman PA, Sikora RA. Endophytes: An emerging tool for biological control. Biological Control. 2008;**46**(1):1-3

[9] Faeth SH. Fungal endophytes: Common host plant symbionts but uncommon mutualists. Integrative and Comparative Biology. 2002;**42**(2):360-368

[10] Chaudhary P, Agri U, Chaudhary A, Kumar A, Kumar G. Endophytes and their potential in biotic stress management and crop production. Frontiers in Microbiology. 2022;**13**:1-2

[11] Gwinn KD. Relationship between endophyte infestation level of tall fescue seed lots and *Rhizoctonia zeae* seedling disease. Plant Disease. 1992;**76**(9):911

[12] Silva DPD, Cardoso MS, Macedo AJ. Endophytic fungi as a source of antibacterial compounds—A focus on gram-negative bacteria. Antibiotics. 2022;**11**(11):1509

[13] Akram S, Ahmed A, He P, He P, Liu Y, Wu Y, et al. Uniting the role of endophytic fungi against plant pathogens and their interaction. Journal of Fungi. 2023;**9**(1):72

[14] Redkar A, Sabale M, Zuccaro A, Di Pietro A. Determinants of endophytic and pathogenic lifestyle in root colonizing fungi. Current Opinion in Plant Biology. 2022;**67**:102226

[15] Kumar KK, Dara SK. Fungal and bacterial endophytes as microbial control agents for plant-parasitic nematodes. International Journal of Environmental Research and Public Health. 2021;**18**(8):4269

[16] Ibiang SR, Usami T, Sakamoto K, Ibiang YB. Lettuce tolerance to verticillium wilt after inoculation with *Penicillium pinophilum* and rhizophagus intraradices. Physiological and Molecular Plant Pathology. 2023;**128**:102171

[17] Song Y, Cui H, Guo W, Sindhu L, Lv S, Li L, et al. Endophytic fungi improved wheat resistance to *Rhopalosiphum padi* by decreasing its feeding efficiency and population fitness. Ecotoxicology and Environmental Safety. 2024;**270**:115865

[18] Terhonen E, Sipari N, Asiegbu FO. Inhibition of phytopathogens by fungal root endophytes of Norway spruce. Biological Control. 2016;**99**:53-63

[19] Xia Y, Liu J, Chen C, Mo X, Tan Q, He Y, et al. The multifunctions and future prospects of endophytes and their metabolites in plant disease management. Microorganisms. 2022;**10**(5):1072

[20] Bamisile BS, Dash CK, Akutse KS, Keppanan R, Wang L. Fungal endophytes: Beyond herbivore management. Frontiers in Microbiology. 2018;**9**:1-11

[21] Sharon O, Sun X, Ezrati S, Kagan-Trushina N, Sharon A. Transmission mode and assembly of seed fungal endophyte communities in wheat and wheat wild relatives. Phytobiomes Journal. 2023;**7**(1):113-124

[22] Gundel PE, Rudgers JA, Ghersa CM. Incorporating the process of vertical transmission into understanding of host–symbiont dynamics. Oikos. 2011;**120**(8):1121-1128

[23] Górzyńska K, Olejniczak P, Węgrzyn E. The fungus clonostachys *Epichloë* alters the influence of the *Epichloë* endophyte on seed germination and the biomass of *Puccinellia distans* grass. Frontiers in Microbiology. 2023;**14**:1-10

[24] Lv H, Li X, He D, Chen X, Liu M, Lan Y, et al. Genotype-controlled vertical transmission exerts selective pressure on community assembly of *salvia miltiorrhiza*. Microbial Ecology. 2023;**86**(4):2934-2948

[25] Hodgson S, de Cates C, Hodgson J, Morley NJ, Sutton BC, Gange AC. Vertical transmission of fungal endophytes is widespread in forbs. Ecology and Evolution. 2014;**4**(8):1199-1208

[26] Zhang W, Forester NT, Moon CD, Maclean PH, Gagic M, Arojju SK, et al. *Epichloë* seed transmission efficiency is influenced by plant defense response mechanisms. Frontiers in Plant Science. 2022;**13**:1-17

[27] Freitas PP, Hampton JG, Phil RM, Glare TR, Miller PP, Card SD. A tale of two grass species: Temperature affects the symbiosis of a mutualistic *Epichloë* endophyte in both tall fescue and perennial ryegrass. Frontiers in Plant Science. 2020;**11**:1-12

[28] Sneck ME, Rudgers JA, Young CA, Miller TEX. Variation in the prevalence and transmission of heritable symbionts across host populations in heterogeneous environments. Microbial Ecology. 2017;**74**(3):640-653

[29] Whitaker BK, Christian N, Chai Q, Clay K. Foliar fungal endophyte community structure is independent of phylogenetic relatedness in an asteraceae common garden. Ecology and Evolution. 2020;**10**(24):13895-13912

[30] Miller JD, Cherid H, Sumarah MW, Adams GW. Horizontal transmission of the *Picea glauca* foliar endophyte *Phialocephala* scopiformis CBS 120377. Fungal Ecology. 2009;**2**(2):98-101

[31] Brentassi ME, Medina R, de la Fuente D, Franco MEE, Toledo AV, Saparrat MCN, et al. Endomycobiome associated with females of the

planthopper *Delphacodes kuscheli* (Hemiptera: Delphacidae): A metabarcoding approach. Heliyon. 2020;**6**(8):e04634

[32] Cardinale M, Schnell S. Is the plant microbiome transmitted from pollen to seeds? Frontiers in Microbiology. 2024;**15**:1-5

[33] Wiewióra B, Żurek G, Pańka D. Is the vertical transmission of neotyphodium lolii in perennial ryegrass the only possible way to the spread of endophytes? PLoS One. 2015;**10**(2):e0117231

[34] Della, Mónica IF, Vignale MV, Scervino JM, Iannone LJ, Novas MV. Role of fungal endophytes on mycorrhizal-plant association and its impact on plant fitness. In: Microbial Endophytes and Plant Growth. Amsterdam, The Netherlands: Elsevier; 2023. pp. 117-136

[35] Bacon CW, Porter JK, Robbins JD, Luttrell ES. *Epichloë* typhina from toxic tall fescue grasses. Applied and Environmental Microbiology. 1977;**34**(5):576-581

[36] Porter JK. Chemical constituents of grass endophytes. In: Biotechnology of Endophytic Fungi of Grasses. Boca Raton, FL: CRC Press; 2018. pp. 103-123

[37] Porter JK. Analysis of endophyte toxins: Fescue and other grasses toxic to livestock. Journal of Animal Science. 1995;**73**(3):871-880

[38] Moubarak AS, Piper EL, West CP, Johnson ZB. Interaction of purified ergovaline from endophyte-infected tall fescue with synaptosomal ATPase enzyme system. Journal of Agricultural and Food Chemistry. 1993;**41**(3):407-409

[39] Thompson FN, Stuedemann JA, Hill NS. Anti-quality factors associated with alkaloids in eastern temperate pasture. Journal of Range Management. 2001;**54**(4):474

[40] Shiba T, Arakawa A, Sugawara K. Effects of alkaloids from fungal endophytes in grass – *Epichloë* associations on survival of the sorghum plant bug (*Stenotus rubrovittatus*). Grassland Science. 2015;**61**(1):24-27

[41] Shiba T, Sugawara K. Fungal loline alkaloids in grass–endophyte associations confer resistance to the rice leaf bug, *Trigonotylus caelestialium*. Entomologia Experimentalis et Applicata. 2009;**130**(1):55-62

[42] Siegel MR, Latch GCM, Bush LP, Fannin FF, Rowan DD, Tapper BA, et al. Fungal endophyte-infected grasses: Alkaloid accumulation and aphid response. Journal of Chemical Ecology. 1990;**16**(12):3301-3315

[43] Bacetty AA, Snook ME, Glenn AE, Noe JP, Hill N, Culbreath A, et al. Toxicity of endophyte-infected tall fescue alkaloids and grass metabolites on *Pratylenchus scribneri*. Phytopathology. 2009;**99**(12):1336-1345

[44] Meyer SLF, Patchett BJ, Gillanders TJ, Kantor MR, Timper P, MacDonald MH. *Festulolium* and fungal endophyte associations: Host status for *Meloidogyne incognita* and nematotoxic plant extracts. Journal of Nematology. 2020;**52**(1):1-16

[45] Shi X, Qin T, Qu Y, Zhang J, Hao G, Zhao Y, et al. Comparative omics analysis of endophyte-infected and endophyte-free *Achnatherum sibiricum* in response to pathogenic fungi. Biological Control. 2022;**175**:105040

[46] Fernando K, Reddy P, Spangenberg GC, Rochfort SJ,

Guthridge KM. Metabolic potential of *Epichloë* endophytes for host grass fungal disease resistance. Microorganisms. 2021;**10**(1):64

[47] Li F, Mei D, Ren T, Song Q. Crude extracts and secondary metabolites of *Epichloë bromicola* against *Phytophthora infestans*. Chemistry and Biodiversity. 2023;**20**(1):1-11

[48] Ju Y, Zhong R, Christensen MJ, Zhang X. Effects of *Epichloë gansuensis* endophyte on the root and rhizosphere soil bacteria of *Achnatherum inebrians* under different moisture conditions. Frontiers in Microbiology. 2020;**11**:1-13

[49] Yang Z, Jin Y, Hou F, Bowatte S. Soil microbial and chemical responses to foliar *Epichloë* fungal infection in *Lolium perenne*, *Hordeum brevisubulatum* and *Achnatherum inebrians*. Fungal Ecology. 2021;**53**:101091

[50] Kumar P, Chaturvedi R, Sundar D, Bisaria VS. *Piriformospora indica* enhances the production of pentacyclic triterpenoids in *Lantana camara L*. suspension cultures. Plant Cell, Tissue and Organ Culture (PCTOC). 2016;**125**(1):23-29

[51] Abdelaziz ME, Kim D, Ali S, Fedoroff NV, Al-Babili S. The endophytic fungus *Piriformospora indica* enhances *Arabidopsis thaliana* growth and modulates Na + /K + homeostasis under salt stress conditions. Plant Science. 2017;**263**:107-115

[52] Lanza M, Haro R, Conchillo LB, Benito B. The endophyte *Serendipita indica* reduces the sodium content of Arabidopsis plants exposed to salt stress: Fungal ENA ATPases are expressed and regulated at high pH and during plant co-cultivation in salinity. Environmental Microbiology. 2019;**21**(9):3364-3378

[53] Wu C, Yang Y, Wang Y, Zhang W, Sun H. Colonization of root endophytic fungus *Serendipita indica* improves drought tolerance of *Pinus taeda* seedlings by regulating metabolome and proteome. Frontiers in Microbiology. 2024;**15**:1-24

[54] Li H, Fu S, Zhu J, Gao W, Chen L, Li X, et al. Nitric oxide generated by *Piriformospora indica* -induced nitrate reductase promotes tobacco growth by regulating root architecture and ammonium and nitrate transporter gene expression. Journal of Plant Interactions. 2022;**17**(1):861-872

[55] Rong ZY, Lei AQ, Wu QS, Srivastava AK, Hashem A, Abd_ Allah EF, et al. *Serendipita indica* promotes P acquisition and growth in tea seedlings under P deficit conditions by increasing cytokinins and indoleacetic acid and phosphate transporter gene expression. Frontiers in Plant Science. 2023;**14**:1-11

[56] Prasad D, Verma N, Bakshi M, Narayan OP, Singh AK, Dua M, et al. Functional characterization of a magnesium transporter of root Endophytic fungus *Piriformospora indica*. Frontiers in Microbiology. 2019;**9**:1-14

[57] Padash A, Shahabivand S, Behtash F, Aghaee A. A practicable method for zinc enrichment in lettuce leaves by the endophyte fungus *Piriformospora indica* under increasing zinc supply. Scientia Horticulturae. 2016;**213**:367-372

[58] Verma N, Narayan OP, Prasad D, Jogawat A, Panwar SL, Dua M, et al. Functional characterization of a high-affinity iron transporter (*PiFTR*) from the endophytic fungus *Piriformospora indica* and its role in plant growth and development. Environmental Microbiology. 2022;**24**(2):689-706

[59] Kaval A, Yılmaz H, Tunca Gedik S, Yıldız Kutman B, Kutman ÜB. The fungal root endophyte *Serendipita indica* (*Piriformospora indica*) enhances bread and durum wheat performance under boron toxicity at both vegetative and generative stages of development through mechanisms unrelated to mineral homeostasis. Biology (Basel). 2023;**12**(8):1098

[60] Shukla J, Mohd S, Kushwaha AS, Narayan S, Saxena PN, Bahadur L, et al. Endophytic fungus *Serendipita indica* reduces arsenic mobilization from root to fruit in colonized tomato plant. Environmental Pollution. 2022;**298**:118830

[61] Shukla J, Narayan S, Mishra A, Shirke PA, Kumar M. Reduction of arsenic accumulation in rice grain by endophytic fungus *Serendipita indica*. Rhizosphere. 2023;**26**:100680

[62] Roylawar P, Khandagale K, Nanda S, Soumia PS, Jadhav S, Mahajan V, et al. Colonization of *Serendipita indica* promotes resistance against *Spodoptera exigua* in onion (*Allium cepa L.*). Frontiers in Microbiology. 2023;**14**:1-11

[63] Chen CY, Huang PH, Yeh KW, Wang SJ. Colonization of *Piriformospora indica* enhances insect herbivore resistance of rice plants through jasmonic acid- and antioxidant-mediated defense mechanisms. Journal of Plant Interactions. 2022;**17**(1):9-18. Available from: https://www.tandfonline.com/doi/abs/10.1080/17429145.2021.2008031

[64] Atia MAM, Abdeldaym EA, Abdelsattar M, Ibrahim DSS, Saleh I, Elwahab MA, et al. *Piriformospora indica* promotes cucumber tolerance against root-knot nematode by modulating photosynthesis and innate responsive genes. Saudi Journal of Biological Sciences. 2020;**27**(1):279-287

[65] Deshmukh SD, Kogel KH. *Piriformospora indica* protects barley from root rot caused by *Fusarium graminearum*. Journal of Plant Diseases and Protection. 2007;**114**(6):263-268

[66] Fakhro A, Andrade-Linares DR, von Bargen S, Bandte M, Büttner C, Grosch R, et al. Impact of *Piriformospora indica* on tomato growth and on interaction with fungal and viral pathogens. Mycorrhiza. 2010;**20**(3):191-200

[67] Chowdhury MZH, Mostofa MG, Mim MF, Haque MA, Karim MA, Sultana R, et al. The fungal endophyte *Metarhizium anisopliae* (MetA1) coordinates salt tolerance mechanisms of rice to enhance growth and yield. Plant Physiology and Biochemistry. 2024;**207**:108328

[68] Xu R, Li T, Cui H, Wang J, Yu X, Ding Y, et al. Diversity and characterization of Cd-tolerant dark septate endophytes (DSEs) associated with the roots of Nepal alder (*Alnus nepalensis*) in a metal mine tailing of Southwest China. Applied Soil Ecology. 2015;**93**:11-18

[69] Su Z, Zeng Y, Li X, Perumal AB, Zhu J, Lu X, et al. The endophytic fungus *Piriformospora Indica*-assisted alleviation of cadmium in tobacco. Journal of Fungi. 2021;**7**(8):675

[70] Ren A, Li C, Gao Y. Endophytic fungus improves growth and metal uptake of *Lolium Arundinaceum* Darbyshire ex. Schreb. International Journal of Phytoremediation. 2011;**13**(3):233-243

[71] George NM, Hany-Ali G, Abdelhaliem E, Abdel-Haleem M. Alleviating the drought stress and improving the plant resistance properties of *Triticum aestivum* via biopriming with

Aspergillus fumigatus. BMC Plant Biology. 2024;**24**(1):150

[72] Bae H, Sicher RC, Kim MS, Kim SH, Strem MD, Melnick RL, et al. The beneficial endophyte *Trichoderma hamatum* isolate DIS 219b promotes growth and delays the onset of the drought response in *Theobroma cacao*. Journal of Experimental Botany. 2009;**60**(11):3279-3295

[73] Yang T, Ma S, Dai CC. Drought degree constrains the beneficial effects of a fungal endophyte on *Atractylodes lancea*. Journal of Applied Microbiology. 2014;**117**(5):1435-1449

[74] Hubbard M, Germida JJ, Vujanovic V. Fungal endophytes enhance wheat heat and drought tolerance in terms of grain yield and second-generation seed viability. Journal of Applied Microbiology. 2014;**116**(1):109-122

[75] Shen J, Chen Y. *Serendipita indica*: A biostimulant enhancing low-temperature tolerance and active constituent levels in *Polygonum cuspidatum*. Agriculture. 2023;**14**(1):7

[76] Hiruma K, Gerlach N, Sacristán S, Nakano RT, Hacquard S, Kracher B, et al. Root endophyte *Colletotrichum tofieldiae* confers plant fitness benefits that are phosphate status dependent. Cell. 2016;**165**(2):464-474

[77] Svietlova N, Reichelt M, Zhyr L, Majumder A, Scholz SS, Grabe V, et al. The beneficial fungus *Mortierella hyalina* modulates amino acid homeostasis in arabidopsis under nitrogen starvation. International Journal of Molecular Sciences. 2023;**24**(22):16128

[78] Suwannarach N, Kumla J, Bussaban B, Lumyong S. Biocontrol of *Rhizoctonia solani* AG-2, the causal agent of damping-off by *Muscodor cinnamomi* CMU-Cib 461. World Journal of Microbiology and Biotechnology. 2012;**28**(11):3171-3177

[79] Gakuubi MM, Munusamy M, Liang ZX, Ng SB. Fungal endophytes: A promising frontier for discovery of novel bioactive compounds. Journal of Fungi. 2021;**7**(10):786

[80] Bhunjun CS, Phukhamsakda C, Hyde KD, McKenzie EHC, Saxena RK, Li Q. Do all fungi have ancestors with endophytic lifestyles? Fungal Diversity. 2023;**125**(1):73-98

[81] Zakaria L, Wan Aziz WN. Molecular identification of endophytic fungi from banana leaves (*Musa spp*.). Tropical Life Sciences Research. 2018;**29**(2):201-211

[82] Sessa L, Abreo E, Lupo S. Diversity of fungal latent pathogens and true endophytes associated with fruit trees in Uruguay. Journal of Phytopathology. 2018;**166**(9):633-647

[83] Cai H, Yu N, Liu Y, Wei X, Guo C. Meta-analysis of fungal plant pathogen *Fusarium oxysporum* infection-related gene profiles using transcriptome datasets. Frontiers in Microbiology. 2022;**13**:1-11

[84] Ekwomadu TI, Akinola SA, Mwanza M. *Fusarium* mycotoxins, their metabolites (free, emerging, and masked), food safety concerns, and health impacts. International Journal of Environmental Research and Public Health. 2021;**18**(22):11741

[85] Xia R, Schaafsma AW, Wu F, Hooker DC. Impact of the improvements in *Fusarium* head blight and agronomic management on economics of winter wheat. World Mycotoxin Journal. 2020;**13**(3):423-440

[86] Okungbowa FI, Shittu HO. *Fusarium* Wilts: An overview. Environmental Research Journal. 2012;**6**(2):84-102

[87] Nefzi A, Ben ARA, Jabnoun-Khiareddine H, Ammar N, Daami-Remadi M. Ability of endophytic fungi associated with *Withania somnifera L.* to control *Fusarium* crown and root rot and to promote growth in tomato. Brazilian Journal of Microbiology. 2019;**50**(2):481-494

[88] Waweru B, Turoop L, Kahangi E, Coyne D, Dubois T. Non-pathogenic *Fusarium oxysporum* endophytes provide field control of nematodes, improving yield of banana (*Musa sp.*). Biological Control. 2014;**74**:82-88

[89] Inderbitzin P, Subbarao KV. *Verticillium* systematics and evolution: How confusion impedes Verticillium wilt management and how to resolve it. Phytopathology. 2014;**104**(6):564-574

[90] Deketelaere S, Spiessens K, Pollet S, Tyvaert L, De RL, Callens D, et al. Towards practical application of *Verticillium isaacii* Vt305 to control Verticillium wilt of cauliflower: Exploring complementary biocontrol strategies. Plants. 2020;**9**(11):1469

[91] Wheeler DL, Dung JKS, Johnson DA. From pathogen to endophyte: An endophytic population of *Verticillium dahliae* evolved from a sympatric pathogenic population. New Phytologist. 2019;**222**(1):497-510

[92] DeMers M. Alternaria alternata as endophyte and pathogen. Microbiology (N Y). 2022;**168**(3):1-15

[93] Díaz-González S, Marín P, Sánchez R, Arribas C, Kruse J, González-Melendi P, et al. Mutualistic fungal endophyte *Colletotrichum tofieldiae* Ct0861 colonizes and increases growth and yield of maize and tomato plants. Agronomy. 2020;**10**(10):1493

[94] Khan MS, Gao J, Munir I, Zhang M, Liu Y, Moe TS, et al. Characterization of Endophytic fungi, *Acremonium sp.*, from *Lilium davidii* and analysis of its antifungal and plant growth-promoting effects. BioMed Research International. 2021;**2021**:1-14

[95] Funk CR, White RH, Breen JP. Importance of *Acremonium* endophytes in turf-grass breeding and management. Agriculture, Ecosystems and Environment. 1993;**44**(1-4):215-232

[96] U'Ren JM, Oita S, Lutzoni F, Miadlikowska J, Ball B, Carbone I, et al. Environmental drivers and cryptic biodiversity hotspots define endophytes in Earth's largest terrestrial biome. Current Biology. 2024;**34**(5):1148-1156.e7

[97] Arnold AE, Maynard Z, Gilbert GS, Coley PD, Kursar TA. Are tropical fungal endophytes hyperdiverse? Ecology Letters. 2000;**3**(4):267-274

[98] Arnold AE, Lutzoni F. Diversity and host range of foliar fungal endophytes: Are tropical leaves biodiversity hotspots? Ecology. 2007;**88**(3):541-549

[99] Zhou YQ, Yao SC, Wang J, Xie XY, Tan XM, Huang RS, et al. Cultivable endophytic fungal community associated with the karst endemic plant nervilia fordii and their antimicrobial activity. Frontiers in Microbiology. 2022;**13**:1-15

[100] Vidal A, Parada R, Mendoza L, Cotoras M. Endophytic fungi isolated from plants growing in central andean precordillera of Chile with antifungal activity against botrytis cinerea. Journal of Fungi. 2020;**6**(3):149

[101] Zachow C, Berg C, Müller H, Meincke R, Komon-Zelazowska M, Druzhinina IS, et al. Fungal diversity in the rhizosphere of endemic plant species of Tenerife (Canary Islands): Relationship to vegetation zones and environmental factors. The ISME Journal. 2009;**3**(1):79-92

[102] Jin H, Yan Z, Liu Q, Yang X, Chen J, Qin B. Diversity and dynamics of fungal endophytes in leaves, stems and roots of *Stellera chamaejasme L.* in northwestern China. Antonie Van Leeuwenhoek. 2013;**104**(6):949-963

[103] Gao Y, Li Z, Han Y. Community structure of endophytic fungi in roots and leaves of fagopyrum mill and *Avena sativa* in a Chinese northern cold region. Bioscience Journal. 2023;**39**:e39039

[104] Zuo Y, Li X, Yang J, Liu J, Zhao L, He X. Fungal endophytic community and diversity associated with desert shrubs driven by plant identity and organ differentiation in extremely arid desert ecosystem. Journal of Fungi. 2021;**7**(7):578

[105] Zhou J, Li X, Huang PW, Dai CC. Endophytism or saprophytism: Decoding the lifestyle transition of the generalist fungus phomopsis liquidambari. Microbiological Research. 2018;**206**:99-112

[106] Stone JK, Polishook JD, White JF. Endophytic fungi. In: Biodiversity of Fungi: Inventory and Monitoring Methods. Burlington, MA: Elsevier Academic Press; 2004. pp. 241-270

[107] Wang S, Ma T, Yao X, Yao Z, Wang Z, Dong Z, et al. Structure of endophytes in the root, stem, and leaf tissues of sweetpotato and their response to sweetpotato scab disease caused by elsinoë batatas. Agronomy. 2023;**13**(12):2965

[108] Khare E, Mishra J, Arora NK. Multifaceted interactions between endophytes and plant: Developments and prospects. Frontiers in Microbiology. 2018;**9**:1-12

[109] Bastías DA, Alejandra Martínez-Ghersa M, Newman JA, Card SD, Mace WJ, Gundel PE. The plant hormone salicylic acid interacts with the mechanism of anti-herbivory conferred by fungal endophytes in grasses. Plant, Cell and Environment. 2018;**41**(2):395-405

[110] Di X, Takken FLW, Tintor N. How phytohormones shape interactions between plants and the soil-borne fungus *Fusarium oxysporum*. Frontiers in Plant Science. 2016;7:1-9

[111] González-Guzmán A, Rey MD, Froussart E, Quesada-Moraga E. Elucidating the effect of endophytic entomopathogenic fungi on bread wheat growth through signaling of immune response-related hormones. Applied and Environmental Microbiology. 2022;**88**(18):1-15

[112] Schardl CL, Leuchtmann A, Spiering MJ. Symbioses of grasses with seedborne fungal endophytes. Annual Review of Plant Biology. 2004;**55**(1):315-340

[113] Dupont P, Eaton CJ, Wargent JJ, Fechtner S, Solomon P, Schmid J, et al. Fungal endophyte infection of ryegrass reprograms host metabolism and alters development. New Phytologist. 2015;**208**(4):1227-1240

[114] Zuccaro A, Lahrmann U, Güldener U, Langen G, Pfiffi S, Biedenkopf D, et al. Endophytic life strategies decoded by genome and transcriptome analyses of the mutualistic root symbiont *Piriformospora indica*. PLoS Pathogens. 2011;**7**(10):e1002290

[115] Jing M, Xu X, Peng J, Li C, Zhang H, Lian C, et al. Comparative genomics of three aspergillus strains reveals insights into endophytic lifestyle and endophyte-induced plant growth promotion. Journal of Fungi. 2022;**8**(7):690

[116] Eaton CJ, Dupont PY, Solomon P, Clayton W, Scott B, Cox MP. A Core gene set describes the molecular basis of mutualism and antagonism in *Epichloë* spp. Molecular Plant-Microbe Interactions®. 2015;**28**(3):218-231

[117] Yan D, Cai N, Nong X, Wang G, Wang Q, Ullah H, et al. Transcriptomic differences in response to *Metarhizium anisopliae* and *Trichoderma harzianum* uncovers major regulative genes and pathways for establishment of beneficial relationship in peanut. Biological Control. 2022;**172**:104964

[118] Hu S, Bidochka MJ. Abscisic acid implicated in differential plant responses of *Phaseolus vulgaris* during endophytic colonization by metarhizium and pathogenic colonization by *Fusarium*. Scientific Reports. 2021;**11**(1):11327

[119] Mathew SA, Helander M, Saikkonen K, Vankova R, Dobrev PI, Dirihan S, et al. Epichloë endophytes shape the foliar endophytic fungal microbiome and Alter the auxin and salicylic acid phytohormone levels in two meadow fescue cultivars. Journal of Fungi. 2023;**9**(1):90

[120] Ma LJ, van der Does HC, Borkovich KA, Coleman JJ, Daboussi MJ, Di Pietro A, et al. Comparative genomics reveals mobile pathogenicity chromosomes in *Fusarium*. Nature. 2010;**464**(7287):367-373

[121] Wei H, Zhong Z, Li Z, Zhang Y, Stukenbrock EH, Tang B, et al. Loss of the accessory chromosome converts a pathogenic tree-root fungus into a mutualistic endophyte. Plant Communications. 2024;**5**(1):100672

[122] Arnold BJ, Huang IT, Hanage WP. Horizontal gene transfer and adaptive evolution in bacteria. Nature Reviews. Microbiology. 2022;**20**(4):206-218

[123] Glenn AE, Davis CB, Gao M, Gold SE, Mitchell TR, Proctor RH, et al. Two horizontally transferred xenobiotic resistance gene clusters associated with detoxification of benzoxazolinones by *Fusarium* species. PLoS One. 2016;**11**(1):e0147486

[124] Gao S, Gold SE, Wisecaver JH, Zhang Y, Guo L, Ma LJ, et al. Genome-wide analysis of *Fusarium* verticillioides reveals inter-kingdom contribution of horizontal gene transfer to the expansion of metabolism. Fungal Genetics and Biology. 2019;**128**:60-73

[125] Zhou L, Li X, Kotta-Loizou I, Dong K, Li S, Ni D, et al. A mycovirus modulates the endophytic and pathogenic traits of a plant associated fungus. The ISME Journal. 2021;**15**(7):1893-1906

[126] Pedersen C, Marzano SYL. Mechanisms of primed Defense: Plant immunity induced by endophytic colonization of a mycovirus-induced hypovirulent fungal pathogen. Molecular Plant-Microbe Interactions®. 2023;**36**(11):726-736

[127] Stierle A, Strobel G, Stierle D. Taxol and taxane production by *Taxomyces andreanae*, an endophytic fungus of pacific yew. Science (1979). 1993;**260**(5105):214-216

[128] Staniek A, Woerdenbag HJ, Kayser O. Endophytes: Exploiting biodiversity for the improvement of natural product-based drug

discovery. Journal of Plant Interactions. 2008;**3**(2):75-93

[129] Yang Y, Zhao H, Barrero RA, Zhang B, Sun G, Wilson IW, et al. Genome sequencing and analysis of the paclitaxel-producing endophytic fungus *Penicillium aurantiogriseum* NRRL 62431. BMC Genomics. 2014;**15**(1):69

[130] Shinozuka H, Hettiarachchige IK, Shinozuka M, Cogan NOI, Spangenberg GC, Cocks BG, et al. Horizontal transfer of a ß-1,6-glucanase gene from an ancestral species of fungal endophyte to a cool-season grass host. Scientific Reports. 2017;**7**(1):9024

[131] Wang H, Sun S, Ge W, Zhao L, Hou B, Wang K, et al. Horizontal gene transfer of *Fhb7* from fungus underlies *Fusarium* head blight resistance in wheat. Science (1979). 2020;**368**(6493):1-7

[132] Yin H, Sun YH. Vincamine-producing endophytic fungus isolated from *Vinca* minor. Phytomedicine. 2011;**18**(8-9):802-805

[133] Yin H, Zhao Q, Sun FM, An T. Gentiopicrin-producing endophytic fungus isolated from gentiana macrophylla. Phytomedicine. 2009;**16**(8):793-797

[134] Hebert PDN, Cywinska A, Ball SL, deWaard JR. Biological identifications through DNA barcodes. Proceedings of the Royal Society of London - Series B: Biological Sciences. 2003;**270**(1512):313-321

[135] Waheeda K, Shyam KV. Formulation of novel surface sterilization method and culture media for the isolation of endophytic actinomycetes from medicinal plants and its antibacterial activity. Journal of Plant Pathology and Microbiology. 2017;**08**(02):1-9

[136] Saldierna Guzmán JP, Nguyen K, Hart SC. Simple methods to remove microbes from leaf surfaces. Journal of Basic Microbiology. 2020;**60**(8):730-734

[137] Collado J, Platas G, Paulus B, Bills GF. High-throughput culturing of fungi from plant litter by a dilution-to-extinction technique. FEMS Microbiology Ecology. 2007;**60**(3):521-533

[138] Donegan KK, Schaller DL, Stone JK, Ganio LM, Reed G, Hamm PB, et al. Microbial populations, fungal species diversity and plant pathogen levels in field plots of potato plants expressing the bacillus thuringiensis var. tenebrionis endotoxin. Transgenic Research. 1996;**5**(1):25-35

[139] Bills GF, Polishook JD. Abundance and diversity of microfungi in leaf litter of a lowland rain forest in Costa Rica. Mycologia. 1994;**86**(2):187

[140] Lundberg DS, Lebeis SL, Paredes SH, Yourstone S, Gehring J, Malfatti S, et al. Defining the core *Arabidopsis thaliana* root microbiome. Nature. 2012;**488**(7409):86-90

[141] Khan AL, Al-Harrasi A, Al-Rawahi A, Al-Farsi Z, Al-Mamari A, Waqas M, et al. Endophytic fungi from frankincense tree improves host growth and produces extracellular enzymes and indole acetic acid. PLoS One. 2016;**11**(6):e0158207

[142] Chand K, Shah S, Sharma J, Paudel MR, Pant B. Isolation, characterization, and plant growth-promoting activities of endophytic fungi from a wild orchid *Vanda cristata*. Plant Signaling & Behavior. 2020;**15**(5):1744294

[143] Gong A, Zhou T, Xiao C, Jiang W, Zhou Y, Zhang J, et al. Association

between dipsacus saponin VI level and diversity of endophytic fungi in roots of *Dipsacus asperoides*. World Journal of Microbiology and Biotechnology. 2019;**35**(3):42

[144] Stajich JE, Berbee ML, Blackwell M, Hibbett DS, James TY, Spatafora JW, et al. The fungi. Current Biology. 2009;**19**(18):R840-R845

[145] Gonzalez Garcia V, Portal Onco MA, Rubio SV, Review. Biology and systematics of the form genus *Rhizoctonia*. Spanish Journal of Agricultural Research. 2006;**4**(1):55-79

[146] Uppala SS, Zhou XG, Liu B, Wu M. Plant-based culture media for improved growth and sporulation of *Cercospora janseana*. Plant Disease. 2019;**103**(3):504-508

[147] Leach CM. Sporulation of diverse species of fungi under near-ultraviolet radiation. Canadian Journal of Botany. 1962;**40**(1):151-161

[148] Raja HA, Miller AN, Pearce CJ, Oberlies NH. Fungal identification using molecular tools: A primer for the natural products research community. Journal of Natural Products. 2017;**80**(3):756-770

[149] Taylor JW, Hibbett DS. Toward sequence-based classification of fungal species. IMA Fungus. 2013;**4**(2):A33-A34

[150] Kuhls K, Lieckfeldt E, Samuels GJ, Kovacs W, Meyer W, Petrini O, et al. Molecular evidence that the asexual industrial fungus *Trichoderma reesei* is a clonal derivative of the ascomycete Hypocrea jecorina. National Academy of Sciences of the United States of America. 1996;**93**(15):7755-7760

[151] Chen J, Moinard M, Xu J, Wang S, Foulongne-Oriol M, Zhao R, et al. Genetic analyses of the internal transcribed spacer sequences suggest introgression and duplication in the medicinal mushroom *Agaricus subrufescens*. PLoS One. 2016;**11**(5):e0156250

[152] Stadler M, Lambert C, Wibberg D, Kalinowski J, Cox RJ, Kolařík M, et al. Intragenomic polymorphisms in the ITS region of high-quality genomes of the hypoxylaceae (xylariales, ascomycota). Mycological Progress. 2020;**19**(3):235-245

[153] Blackwell M. The fungi: 1, 2, 3 ... 5.1 million species? American Journal of Botany. 2011;**98**(3):426-438

[154] de Hoog GS, Dukik K, Monod M, Packeu A, Stubbe D, Hendrickx M, et al. Toward a novel multilocus phylogenetic taxonomy for the dermatophytes. Mycopathologia. 2017;**182**(1-2):5-31

[155] Sahoo RK, Gaur M, Subudhi E. Function profiling of microbial community. In: New and Future Developments in Microbial Biotechnology and Bioengineering. Amsterdam, The Netherlands: Elsevier; 2019. pp. 77-85

[156] Verma V, Srivastava A, Garg SK, Singh VP, Arora PK. Incorporating omics-based tools into endophytic fungal research. Biotechnology Notes. 2024;**5**:1-7

[157] Blaxter M, Mann J, Chapman T, Thomas F, Whitton C, Floyd R, et al. Defining operational taxonomic units using DNA barcode data. Philosophical Transactions of the Royal Society B: Biological Sciences. 2005;**360**(1462):1935-1943

[158] Durazzi F, Sala C, Castellani G, Manfreda G, Remondini D, De Cesare A. Comparison between 16S rRNA and shotgun sequencing data

for the taxonomic characterization of the gut microbiota. Scientific Reports. 2021;**11**(1):3030

[159] Adeleke BS, Muller D, Babalola OO. A metagenomic lens into endosphere microbial communities, promises, and discoveries. Letters in Applied Microbiology. 2023;**76**(2):1-10

[160] Coelho LP, Alves R, del Río ÁR, Myers PN, Cantalapiedra CP, Giner-Lamia J, et al. Towards the biogeography of prokaryotic genes. Nature. 2022;**601**(7892):252-256

[161] Rodríguez del Río Á, Giner-Lamia J, Cantalapiedra CP, Botas J, Deng Z, Hernández-Plaza A, et al. Functional and evolutionary significance of unknown genes from uncultivated taxa. Nature. 2024;**626**(7998):377-384

[162] Fadiji AE, Babalola OO. Metagenomics methods for the study of plant-associated microbial communities: A review. Journal of Microbiological Methods. 2020;**170**:105860

[163] Sagita R, Quax WJ, Haslinger K. Current state and future directions of genetics and genomics of endophytic fungi for bioprospecting efforts. Frontiers in Bioengineering and Biotechnology. 2021;**9**:1-26

[164] Li B, Tang M, Tang K, Zhao L, Guo S. Screening for differentially expressed genes in *Anoectochilus roxburghii* (Orchidaceae) during symbiosis with the mycorrhizal fungus *Epulorhiza sp*. Science China. Life Sciences. 2012;**55**(2):164-171

[165] Guo L, Yu H, Wang B, Vescio K, DeIulio GA, Yang H, et al. Metatranscriptomic comparison of endophytic and pathogenic *Fusarium—Arabidopsis* interactions reveals plant transcriptional plasticity. Molecular Plant-Microbe Interactions®. 2021;**34**(9):1071-1083

[166] Bastias DA, Martínez-Ghersa MA, Ballaré CL, Gundel PE. Epichloë fungal endophytes and plant defenses: Not just alkaloids. Trends in Plant Science. 2017;**22**(11):939-948

[167] Constantin ME, de Lamo FJ, Vlieger BV, Rep M, Takken FLW. Endophyte-mediated resistance in tomato to *Fusarium oxysporum* is independent of ET, JA, and SA. Frontiers in Plant Science. 2019;**10**:1-14

[168] Sarkar D, Rovenich H, Jeena G, Nizam S, Tissier A, Balcke GU, et al. The inconspicuous gatekeeper: Endophytic *Serendipita vermifera* acts as extended plant protection barrier in the rhizosphere. New Phytologist. 2019;**224**(2):886-901

[169] Doni F, Fathurrahman F, Mispan MS, Suhaimi NSM, Yusoff WMW, Uphoff N. Transcriptomic profiling of rice seedlings inoculated with the symbiotic fungus *Trichoderma asperellum* SL2. Journal of Plant Growth Regulation. 2019;**38**(4):1507-1515

[170] Saini P, Verma A, Tiwari H, Mishra V, Gautam V. Omics-based approaches in studying fungal endophytes and their associated secondary metabolites. Cham, Switzerland: Springer; 2024. pp. 209-227

[171] Tiwari P, Bae H. Endophytic fungi: Key insights, emerging prospects, and challenges in natural product drug discovery. Microorganisms. 2022;**10**(2):360

[172] Kharwar RN, Sharma VK, Mishra A, Kumar J, Singh DK, Verma SK, et al. Harnessing the phytotherapeutic treasure troves of the ancient medicinal plant *Azadirachta indica* (neem) and

associated endophytic microorganisms. Planta Medica. 2020;**86**(13/14):906-940

[173] Chu LL, Huy NQ, Tung NH. Microorganisms for ginsenosides biosynthesis: Recent progress, challenges, and perspectives. Molecules. 2023;**28**(3):1437

[174] Tiwari P, Thakkar S, Dufossé L. Antimicrobials from endophytes as novel therapeutics to counter drug-resistant pathogens. Critical Reviews in Biotechnology. 2024:1-27

[175] Deshmukh SK, Dufossé L, Chhipa H, Saxena S, Mahajan GB, Gupta MK. Fungal endophytes: A potential source of antibacterial compounds. Journal of Fungi. 2022;**8**(2):164

[176] Caruso DJ, Palombo EA, Moulton SE, Zaferanloo B. Exploring the promise of endophytic fungi: A review of novel antimicrobial compounds. Microorganisms. 2022;**10**(10):1990

[177] Rai N, Gupta P, Keshri PK, Verma A, Mishra P, Kumar D, et al. Fungal endophytes: An accessible source of bioactive compounds with potential anticancer activity. Applied Biochemistry and Biotechnology. 2022;**194**(7):3296-3319

[178] Eshboev F, Mamadalieva N, Nazarov P, Hussain H, Katanaev V, Egamberdieva D, et al. Antimicrobial action mechanisms of natural compounds isolated from endophytic microorganisms. Antibiotics. 2024;**13**(3):271

[179] Tyagi G, Kapoor N, Chandra G, Gambhir L. Cure lies in nature: Medicinal plants and endophytic fungi in curbing cancer. 3 Biotech. 2021;**11**(6):263

[180] Hridoy M, Gorapi MZH, Noor S, Chowdhury NS, Rahman MM, Muscari I, et al. Putative anticancer compounds from plant-derived endophytic fungi: A review. Molecules. 2022;**27**(1):296

[181] Nzimande B, Makhwitine JP, Mkhwanazi NP, Ndlovu SI. Developments in exploring fungal secondary metabolites as antiviral compounds and advances in HIV-1 inhibitor screening assays. Viruses. 2023;**15**(5):1039

[182] Agrawal S, Samanta S, Deshmukh SK. The antidiabetic potential of endophytic fungi: Future prospects as therapeutic agents. Biotechnology and Applied Biochemistry. 2022;**69**(3):1159-1165

[183] Hzounda Fokou JB, Dize D, Etame Loe GM, MHJ N'k, Ngene JP, Ngoule CC, et al. Anti-leishmanial and anti-trypanosomal natural products from endophytes. Parasitology Research. 2021;**120**(3):785-796

[184] Morales-Quintana L, Miño R, Mendez-Yañez A, Gundel PE, Ramos P. Do fungal-endosymbionts improve crop nutritional quality and tolerance to stress by boosting flavonoid-mediated responses? Food Research International. 2022;**161**:111850

[185] Sharma A, Kaushik N, Sharma A, Marzouk T, Djébali N. Exploring the potential of endophytes and their metabolites for bio-control activity. 3 Biotech. 2022;**12**(10):277

[186] Sharma I, Raina A, Choudhary M, Apra KS, Dhar MK. Fungal endophyte bioinoculants as a green alternative towards sustainable agriculture. Heliyon. 2023;**9**(9):e19487

[187] Agrawal S, Bhatt A. Microbial endophytes: Emerging trends and biotechnological applications. Current Microbiology. 2023;**80**(8):249

[188] Dwibedi V, Rath SK, Joshi M, Kaur R, Kaur G, Singh D, et al. Microbial endophytes: Application towards sustainable agriculture and food security. Applied Microbiology and Biotechnology. 2022;**106**(17):5359-5384

[189] Berestetskiy A, Hu Q. The chemical ecology approach to reveal fungal metabolites for arthropod pest management. Microorganisms. 2021;**9**(7):1379

[190] Xu K, Li XQ, Zhao DL, Zhang P. Antifungal secondary metabolites produced by the fungal endophytes: Chemical diversity and potential use in the development of biopesticides. Frontiers in Microbiology. 2021;**12**:1-17

[191] Meena H, Hnamte S, Siddhardha B. Secondary Metabolites from Endophytic Fungi: Chemical Diversity and Application. Cham, Switzerland: Springer; 2019. pp. 145-169

[192] He XJ, Jiao J, Gai QY, Fu JX, Fu YJ, Zhang ZY, et al. Bioprocessing of pigeon pea roots by a novel endophytic fungus *Penicillium rubens* for the improvement of genistein yield using semi-solid-state fermentation with water. Innovative Food Science and Emerging Technologies. 2023;**90**:103519

[193] Li P, Ling X, Zhao S, Xu L, Wang R. Diversity and isolation of endophytic fungi in *Panax japonicus* and biotransformation activity on saponins. Current Pharmaceutical Biotechnology. 2024;**25**(9):1199-1208

[194] Küçüksolak M, Üner G, Ballar Kırmızıbayrak P, Bedir E. Neuroprotective metabolites via fungal biotransformation of a novel sapogenin, cyclocephagenol. Scientific Reports. 2022;**12**(1):18481

[195] Chen Y, Yu D, Huo J, Huang N, Zhang M, Du X. Studies on biotransformation mechanism of *Fusarium sp*. C39 to enhance saponin content of paridis rhizoma. Frontiers in Microbiology. 2022;**13**:1-19

[196] Khare E, Vishwakarma A, Maurya V, Kaistha SD. Endophytic fungi from parasitic-plant cuscuta, and their potential for producing L-asparaginase of pharmaceutical significance. Environmental Sustainability. 2024;**7**(1):93-101

[197] Núñez-García IC, Martínez-Ávila GCG, González-Herrera SM, Tafolla-Arellano JC, Rutiaga-Quiñones OM. Bioprospecting of endophytic fungi from semidesert candelilla (*Euphorbia antisyphilitica Zucc*): Potential for extracellular enzyme production. Journal of Basic Microbiology. 2024;**64**(7):1-13

[198] Hoyos LV, Chaves A, Grandezz D, Medina A, Correa J, Ramirez-Castrillon M, et al. Systematic screening strategy for fungal laccase activity of endophytes from otoba gracilipes with bioremediation potential. Fungal Biology. 2023;**127**(9):1298-1311

[199] González Álvarez Á, Martinez i Quer A, Ellegaard-Jensen L, Sapkota R, Carvalho PN, Johansen A. Fungal removal of cyanotoxins in constructed wetlands: The forgotten degraders. Science of the Total Environment. 2024;**929**:172590

[200] Bonatti E, dos Santos A, Birolli WG, Rodrigues-Filho E. Endophytic, extremophilic and entomophilic fungi strains biodegrade anthracene showing potential for bioremediation. World Journal of Microbiology and Biotechnology. 2023;**39**(6):152

[201] Conceição JCS, Alvarega AD, Mercante LA, Correa DS, Silva EO. Endophytic fungus from handroanthus

impetiginosus immobilized on electrospun nanofibrous membrane for bioremoval of bisphenol A. World Journal of Microbiology and Biotechnology. 2023;**39**(10):261

[202] Marfuah DS, Hamim H, Sulistyaningsih YC, Surono S, Setyaningsih L, Saprudin D. Dark septate endophyte inoculation improved Pb phytoremediation of *Jatropha curcas* and *Reutealis trisperma* on gold mine tailings. Bioremediation Journal. 2023:1-18

[203] de Almeida TT, Tschoeke BAP, Quecine MC, Tezzoto T, Gaziola SA, Azevedo RA, et al. Mechanisms of *Mucor sp*. CM3 isolated from the aquatic macrophyte *Eichhornia crassipes* (Mart.) Solms to increase cadmium bioremediation. Environmental Science and Pollution Research. 2023;**30**(41):93846-93861

[204] Lu Y, Liu T, Bai R, Jia Y, Chen W, Zhao J, et al. Potential application of grape endophytic fungus (alternaria alternata MG1) as bio-adjunct and immobilization carrier of *S. cerevisiae* in improving aroma quality, polyphenol profiles, antioxidant activity and color stability of merlot red wine. LWT. 2024;**198**:116034

Chapter 4

Importance and Applications of Endophytic Fungi

Mostafa Ebadi and Ali Ebadi

Abstract

Endophytic fungi are microorganisms that live symbiotically in healthy plant tissues for all or part of their life cycle without causing disease. They exhibit high biological diversity and have been found in a wide range of plant groups, including both vascular and nonvascular plants. Isolating and identifying endophytic fungi is crucial for studying the evolutionary relationship between plants and fungi. Alongside morphological identification, molecular phylogeny methods are essential for accurately determining fungal species. The ITS region is a crucial molecular marker with a high accuracy rate for identification. Endophytic fungi can enhance plant performance through various mechanisms, including promoting growth, nutrient uptake, and stress tolerance, such as drought and salinity. Fungi play a crucial role in enhancing plant health by promoting growth and increasing resistance to pathogens, insects, and herbivores through the production of secondary metabolites and induction of phytoalexins. These fungi are being explored as a promising source of bioactive compounds with various applications in the pharmaceuticals, food, and agriculture industries.

Keywords: mycelium, ITS, symbiosis, stressors, biological potential

1. Introduction

The term endophyte is derived from the Greek words "endon" meaning within, and "phyte" meaning plant. First introduced in 1866 by Bary, it has been widely used for any type of organism that exists within plant tissues. However, in today's definition, endophytes are organisms that live inside the healthy tissues of plants in a symbiotic relationship without causing disease, either entirely or at least in part [1]. Various organisms, such as fungi, bacteria, and actinomycetes, have been reported as endophytes in plant tissues. Generally, research shows that in most natural ecosystems, plants have a symbiotic relationship with endophytic fungi and mycorrhizae. Unlike mycorrhizal fungi, which colonize plant roots and grow in the rhizosphere region, endophytic fungi are found not only in roots but also in stems and leaves as hyphae in intercellular fluids of tissues. Fossils dating back 400 million years indicate the relationship between plants and endophytes. In this regard, Krings et al. were able to demonstrate the presence of three endophytic fungi inside the plant *Nothia aphylla* Lyon ex El-Saadawy and Lacy by studying thin sections of the fossil related to the plant [2].

Environmental factors, such as rainfall and atmospheric humidity, can influence the presence of some endophytic fungal species. Chareprasert et al. identified that the number of isolates obtained from plants is significantly lower during the dry season [3]. Rodriguez suggested that the low number of isolates during the dry season may be related to the water stress effect on plants [4]. Under water stress, the accumulation of nonstructural carbohydrates in plants occurs, leading to the production of carbon-based defensive compounds, such as tannins, ultimately making it difficult for plants to establish a symbiotic relationship with endophytic fungi during the dry season. However, multiple studies also show the positive impact of endophytic fungi on water stress by increasing biomass production, reducing stomatal conductance, and reducing water loss.

2. Biodiversity of endophytic fungi

Endophytic fungi are highly diverse and can be found in various habitats, such as hot deserts, polar regions, mangroves, forests, and tropical and temperate grasslands. They have been isolated from different plant groups, including grasses, ferns, sedges, and dicots. Previous studies have shown that approximately 3000 different plant species host at least one or more endophytic fungi [5]. In general, *Alternaria* Nees, *Colletotrichum* Corda, *Fusarium* Link, *Gibberella*, *Glomerella*, *Guignardia* Viala and Ravaz, *Leptosphaerulina* McAlpine, *Nigrospora* Zimm., *Phoma* Saccardo, *Phomopsis* Sacc and Roum., and *Xylaria* Hill ex Schrank are the most common genera that have been isolated so far. Additionally, endophytic fungi belonging to the Ascomycota, Basidiomycota, and Zygomycota or Oomycota are the most commonly reported. However, Ascomycota are predominant compared to other groups.

2.1 Classification and taxonomic position of endophytic fungi

Endophytic fungi are divided into two major groups based on taxonomic position, host range, colonization pattern, and ecological function: C-endophytes (*Clavicipitaceous*) and NC-endophytes (*Nonclavicipitaceous*) [6].

C-endophytic fungi belong to the family Clavicipitaceae, order Hypocerales, and phylum Ascomycota. They include species that are saprophytic, insect-associated, and symbiotic with plants such as grasses like fescues and ryegrasses. Most species in this family have the ability to produce alkaloids that are toxic to humans and animals. There are hypotheses suggesting a link between toxicity in animals fed on plants symbiotic with endophytic fungi. Studies by Bacon et al. showed that summer toxicity in livestock fed on *Festuca arundinacea* Schreb. is caused by the presence of the endophytic fungus *Neotyphodium coenophialum* and its alkaloid production [7].

Mycelium C-endophytes are found in intercellular spaces of the leaf sheath, stem, rhizome, and leaf blade. The effects of C-endophytes on the host plant include insect repellency, herbivore deterrence, nematode reduction, increased host resistance to diseases, as well as improvement or enhancement of the host plant's ecophysiological response to non-biological stresses such as drought and metal pollution [8–11].

Most species of NC-endophytes belong to the Ascomycota and, rarely, Basidiomycota branches and are found as symbionts in the leaves of deciduous trees, the aerial parts of grasses, sedges, legumes, and woody and herbaceous plants in various biomes. The effects of NC-endophytes on the host plant include reducing environmental stresses, aiding in host adaptation, increasing biomass, and protecting the host against pathogenic fungi by producing metabolites and inducing defense systems [12–14].

Some researchers have classified endophytes into systemic and nonsystemic endophytes based on the lifestyle of endophytes. Nonsystemic endophytes have short-term relationships with plants, which are optional and temporary, and the population size and species richness of these endophytes over time depend on host factors such as plant growth stage, environmental conditions, and other biological factors, such as pathogens. These endophytes can transition from symbionts to parasites and, in a way, harm the host. On the other hand, systemic endophytes have long-term relationships with plants and have evolved with their plant hosts over time. These endophytes do not harm the host over plant generations, and some of these endophytes that have colonized their host may form part of the plant's endobiome core [15].

Endophytes are also classified into two groups based on the type of plant colonization: obligatory endophytes and facultative endophytes. Obligatory endophytes require the metabolic activity of the plant for their survival and are transmitted through seeds, meaning their origin is not the rhizosphere. On the other hand, facultative endophytes are soil-borne and can colonize the host plant at certain stages of their life cycle. This colonization process occurs through the rhizosphere. After colonization, the organism's survival is influenced by biotic and abiotic factors. This survival is positively correlated with soil physicochemical parameters, organic matter content, and nitrogen. As a result, after rhizosphere colonization, endophytes proliferate in the plant's internal tissues, creating more stable and protected strains in these spaces. The colonization capacity of endophytic microorganisms and resource allocation inside the plant are factors that influence endophyte distribution. Therefore, different plant tissues may have different compositions of endophyte communities [16].

3. Endophyte colonization mechanisms

Successful endophyte colonization requires a high potential to reach the host plant rhizosphere, enter internal tissues, spread within the plant, and overcome the plant's immunity. Successful colonization by endophytes depends on various factors, such as the type of tissue and age of the host plant, the genotype of the host plant, the diversity of endophytic fungal species, and environmental and non-environmental conditions.

The ability of plant components to express their living conditions is a factor that determines the colonization of endophytes. The interaction between fungal endophytes and hosts is controlled at the gene level, involving genes of both partners that are influenced by the environment. The encounter with endophytes by the host plant modulates the level and pattern of gene expression in the host plant.

Endophytic fungi need to pass through the physical barrier of the plant cell wall in order to colonize plant tissues. At the point of contact with a microbe, the plant cell wall undergoes changes that allow the penetration of the plasma membrane and uptake of the microorganism. Endophytic fungi can degrade the plant cell wall by secreting wall-degrading enzymes such as cellulase, laccase, pectinase, and xylanase, altering its structure. As a result, endophytic fungi are trapped in membrane compartments and do not have direct contact with the plant cytoplasm. Molecular exchange between endophytes and plant cytoplasm occurs through their plasma membrane and cell wall, defining a functional interface called the symbiotic interface. The cell wall is involved in the molecular exchange between plants and microorganisms and often mediates the interactions between the plant and microorganisms [17].

4. Isolation and identification of endophytes

Isolation of endophytic fungi is an important step in phylogenetic studies, diversity, interaction with plants, and their application as biofertilizers to improve plant growth and compatibility, as well as to investigate sources of biologically active molecules with industrial and pharmaceutical importance. Isolation involves surface sterilization and placing plant tissue pieces on culture media, followed by the purification of fungi that have grown from the tissues (**Figure 1**).

Identification of fungi at the species level in basic (ecology—taxonomy) and applied (genomics—biological exploration) studies is very important. Identification of endophytic fungi based on morphological characteristics on culture media, such as growth patterns, colony color, tissue, sexual spores, etc., is done using identification keys. However, identifying fungi is difficult due to their high diversity and morphological similarities between different species. Therefore, in addition to the morphological identification of fungi, the use of molecular markers for the accurate identification of fungal species is very important. Species-level identification of fungi is a fundamental part of many research efforts in biological sciences. Taxonomy and phylogenetic systematics are now largely based on phylogenetic trees derived from molecular data. Due to the numerous advantages of molecular data in systematic research, classification based on DNA and DNA barcoding (using long

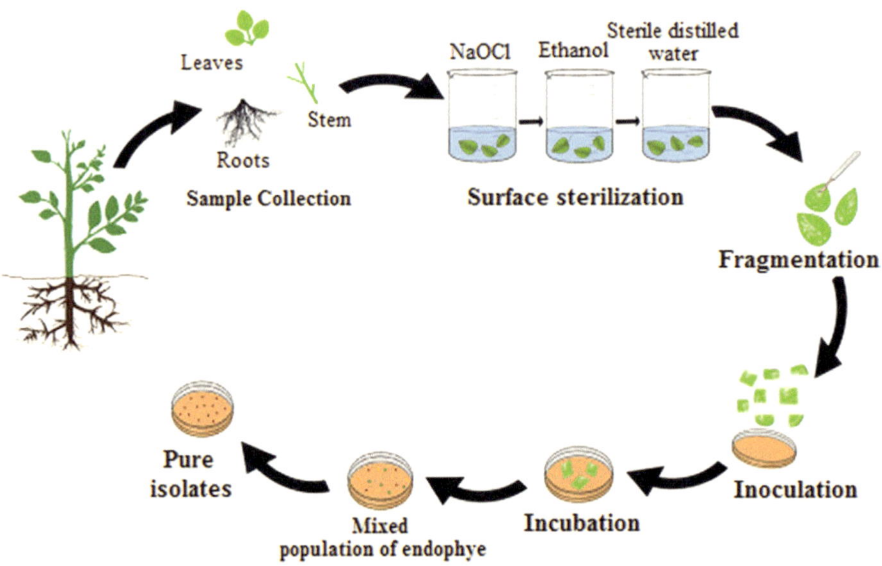

Figure 1.
Isolation of endophytic fungi from different parts of plants [18].

DNA sequences of 500–800 base pairs for species identification) has been explicitly proposed as a tool for species identification [19]. Identification of fungi based on genotype is more reliable because some regions of nucleic acid sequences are very stable and are preserved in a wide range of microorganisms. Studies have shown that specific regions of ribosomal DNA sequences have the highest accuracy for identifying endophytic fungi at the species level and can be used in phylogenetic studies.

In the early 1970s, the use of DNA sequence diversity in evolutionary studies as a tool to assess relationships between organisms began. In the early 1990s, DNA sequences were widely used in evolutionary genetic studies of fungi and populations. The initial acceptance of molecular sequences in fungal studies was mainly due to advances in PCR technologies, DNA sequencing, and the development of a set of fungal DNA primers. By the mid-1990s, polymerase chain reaction (PCR) and DNA sequencing were commonly used in biological laboratories, including for species identification, especially fungal species. These advances have helped to rapidly expand fungal DNA sequences, including multiple DNA fragments from ribosomal RNA gene clusters, in public databases.

Therefore, molecular identification requires the isolation of genomic DNA from fungal strains, PCR amplification of specific DNA sequences using primers, determination of the PCR product sequences in GenBank or other DNA databases, and ultimately retrieval of related sequences from the database and construction of a phylogenetic tree using molecular software.

DNA barcode is a powerful tool for species identification that has the potential to be used for identifying and distinguishing all fungi and overcoming various traditional criteria used to describe different groups of fungi. In 2012, the International Consortium for Fungal Barcoding officially recommended the use of the Internal Transcribed Spacer (ITS) cluster of the nuclear ribosomal RNA gene as the primary fungal barcode. In fungi, the entire ITS region is about 600 base pairs long and includes two variable spacers, ITS-1 and ITS-2 (**Figure 2**). The ITS region is the most common genetic marker for sequencing fungi due to its high variability and is commonly used for addressing research questions related to systematics, phylogeny, and the identification of strains and samples at the species level and below [19].

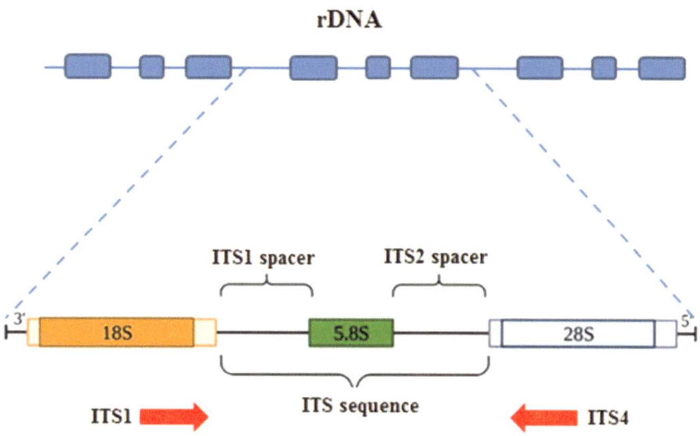

Figure 2.
The nuclear ribosomal internal transcribed spacer (ITS) region. Structure of the rDNA gene in fungi indicating the two regions that were sequenced using ITS1 and ITS4 primers for amplifying ITS (ITS1/5.8S/ITS2) region.

5. The important roles of endophytic fungi for host plant

The interaction between fungi and their hosts leads to changes in the host's metabolism, altered responses to environmental stress, and defense against attackers. Additionally, this interaction results in the production of secondary metabolites by both the fungus and the host, enhancing their ability to respond to the environment [20]. The relationship between fungal endophytes and hosts is controlled at the genetic level, and endophytic fungi have a close interaction with their hosts, facing less competition for space and nutrients and being protected from adverse environmental conditions such as UV light, extreme temperatures, and water scarcity. In return, endophytes improve the growth of their host plants and protect them from biological and non-biological stresses using various mechanisms (**Figure 3**). Physiological adaptations of plants resulting from symbiosis with fungi include the following.

5.1 Increase osmotic regulation

Some endophytes have shown their ability to increase osmotic regulation in plant tissues, which enhances plant resistance to unfavorable conditions such as drought. Often, such strains of endophytes are commercially used in grasslands to help enhance their resistance to stressful conditions [16].

5.2 Oxidative stress regulation

In plants and algae, reactive oxygen species (ROS) are continuously produced as byproducts of some metabolic pathways, including photosynthesis,

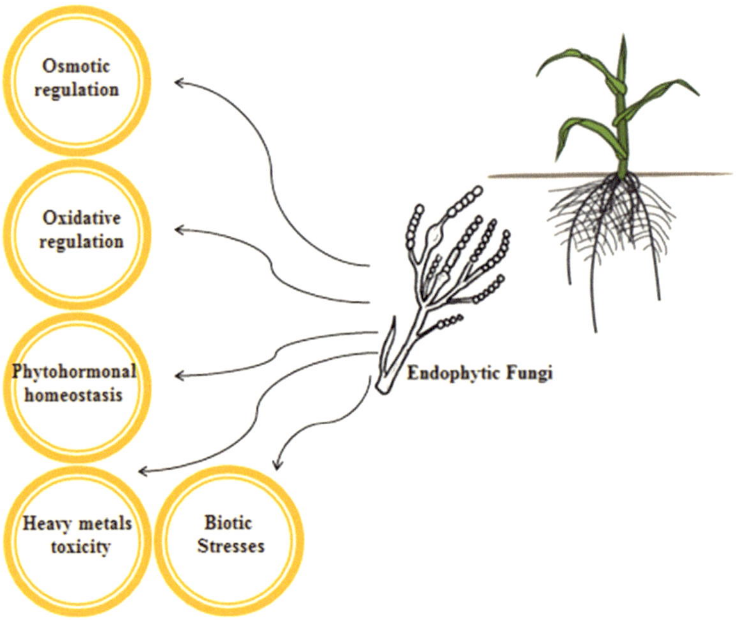

Figure 3.
The physiological roles of endophytic fungi in plants.

light respiration, etc., in various cellular compartments. Different physiological changes occur in plants under stress conditions and sometimes disrupt intracellular and tissue functions. Studies have shown the presence of endophytic fungi to establish redox homeostasis in plants and reduce ROS levels through enzymatic and nonenzymatic antioxidants, enabling host growth under environmental stress conditions. Endophytic fungi induce the production of many antioxidant compounds and enzymes. For example, *Aspergillus flavus* link is an endophytic fungus that has been shown to promote growth in salt-stressed soybeans by controlling antioxidant enzymes such as peroxidase, superoxide dismutase, and catalase. These enzymes can catalyze the detoxification of hydrogen peroxide and superoxide. In addition to enzymatic antioxidants, phenolic acids, flavonoids, carotenoids, tannins, phenolic terpenoids, and glutathione also exhibit antioxidant effects and are regulated by endophytic fungi. These nonenzymatic compounds can neutralize ROS by accepting neutral electrons. Therefore, it can be concluded that endophytic fungi enhance the growth of host plants under non-biological stress conditions [21].

5.3 Phytohormonal homeostasis alteration

Phytohormones are organic compounds that play a role in the growth, physiological processes, and defense mechanisms of plants. Endophytic fungi that interact with plants can alter phytohormonal homeostasis and manipulate physiological responses under environmental stress.

Gibberellic acid (GA) is a phytohormone that controls plant growth and promotes flowering, stem growth, germination, and seed maturation. Many endophytic fungi have biosynthetic pathways for GAs and help improve the performance of host plants by producing active GA.

Abscisic acid (ABA) is a phytohormone that regulates several stress signaling pathways and aids in seed dormancy. The plant's response to stress and reduced plant growth is accompanied by an increase in ABA and a decrease in GA. Under normal conditions, GA has an antagonistic effect with ABA and promotes germination. Gene expression during seed germination is induced by GA signaling, leading to the synthesis of hydrolytic enzymes responsible for breaking down the nutrient reserves in the endosperm of the seed. In this process, endophytic fungi associated with seeds degrade the endosperm, providing a carbon source for seedlings and increasing germination speed.

Many physiological processes such as growth, cell differentiation, germination, formation of vascular tissue, photosynthesis, and root elongation are influenced by the phytohormone auxin (IAA) homeostasis. Some endophytes, especially those colonizing roots, accelerate plant growth by producing IAA. The IAA produced by endophytic fungi is responsible for stimulating root growth, nitrogen uptake, increasing photosynthesis, and promoting host growth under many abiotic stresses. For example, *Phoma glomerata* and *Penicillium* spp. produce biologically active auxins that enhance host growth and nutrient uptake, such as calcium, potassium, and magnesium, under salinity stress.

Salicylic acid (SA) and jasmonic acid (JA) also play important roles in plant defense, which may act synergistically or antagonistically with each other. Various studies have shown that the coexistence of fungal endophytes provides different mechanisms of JA/SA responses [21].

5.4 Heavy metals toxicity

Heavy metals have a significant impact on plants and the ecosystem in which the plant is found. Some metals such as copper, manganese, iron, cobalt, zinc, and chromium are essential for plant metabolism in trace amounts. Plants growing in metal-contaminated areas tend to accumulate them in their cells. These plants usually show altered metabolism and reduced growth rate and biomass production. Phytoremediation is based on the natural ability of plants to extract compounds from the environment. The success of phytoremediation is strongly determined by plant growth and the accumulation of heavy metals in its tissues. Endophytic fungi have the potential to enhance phytoremediation and combat plant toxicity caused by heavy metals in the soil [22]. Endophytic communities play an important role in processing some heavy metals that are toxic to plants. Endophytes reduce environmental stress levels by chelating some toxic metals due to their extensive tolerance mechanism [23]. Many endophytic fungi survive and grow in environments contaminated with toxic metals. The isolation and sequestration of metals outside the cell, metal binding to the cell wall, intracellular complexes, etc., help these fungi to adapt to the toxic environment [22].

Endophytic fungi increase the expression of metal transporters associated with metal flow and distribution inside the plant or improve the plant's antioxidant system and production of plant hormones, leading to increased tolerance of plants to heavy metals [21].

5.5 The role of endophytes in biotic stresses

Endophytic fungi produce bioactive compounds such as alkaloids, quinones, lignans, phenols, etc., which have various medicinal activities including antiviral, antibiotic, anticancer, etc. In addition, recent studies on hydrolytic enzymes produced by endophytic fungi have shown their ability to control plant pathogens. Enzymes such as chitinases, glucanases, proteases, and cellulases can break down structural components of pathogens such as chitin, protein, cellulose, hemicellulose, and DNA [24]. Plant pathogens include fungi, bacteria, insects, and nematodes, and these organisms target plant cells. Endophytes provide these active biological metabolites to plants, helping them defend against pathogens [25, 26]. They are also capable of transferring relevant genes through horizontal gene transfer to the plant genome or vice versa. It is evident that plants without endophytes will be vulnerable to various types of stress and pathogen attacks. Some endophytes produce compounds in plants that reduce herbivory by insects and other herbivores. Fungal endophytes of the Clavicipitaceae family live intercellularly in the aerial parts of plants (such as leaves, stems, and seeds) and produce various alkaloids that deter herbivores. These endophytes are used to increase pest tolerance in commercial forage and turf grasses. It has been shown that *Periglandula* sp. in Convolvolaceae produces ergot alkaloids that make the flowers of these plants highly toxic to herbivores. Similarly, in plants commonly referred to as "Locoweeds" in Fabaceae, *Undifilum* sp. (Pleosporaceae) produces the toxic alkaloid swainsonine, which is a potent anti-herbivore compound and toxin. The examples above demonstrate that endophytes that prevent feeding by pests and insects may be more common than currently documented. Further investigation of fungal endophytes in plants may lead to the discovery of numerous new endophytes that could be used in agricultural products to reduce pest feeding or improve plant tolerance to pests.

6. Industrial application of endophytic fungi

Endophytic fungi are proven sources of secondary metabolites (such as flavonoids, alkaloids, terpenoids, peptides, steroids, phenols, etc.) with potential effects such as anticancer, antibiotic, anti-inflammatory, antioxidant, antiviral, neurotoxic, insecticidal, antifungal, etc. They have various applications in the advancements of biotechnological fields such as pharmaceuticals, agriculture, cosmetics and personal care industries, food industries, and environmental processes [27]. In this regard, the endophytic fungus *Taxomyces andreanae* was isolated from the bark of the Pacific yew tree (*Taxus brevifolia* Nutt.) which has the ability to produce the valuable compound taxol. Many other researchers have also reported and confirmed the biosynthesis of taxol and other secondary metabolites (including vinblastine, vincristine, diosgenin, podophyllotoxin, camptothecin, rohitukine, azadirachtin, piperine, etc.) by fungal endophytes. The following describes some of their applications in various fields.

6.1 Compounds with cytotoxic effects

Cancer is one of the leading causes of death worldwide, with an increasing number of cases reported annually. Taxol was the first reported anticancer drug from endophytic fungi (*Taxomyces andreanae*). Since then, many bioactive metabolites (such as camptothecin, vinblastine, vincristine, podophyllotoxin, rohitukine, piperine, torianic acid, cytochalasins 1–3, cytochalasin E, graphislactone A, butyrolactone, hypericin, ergoflavin, emodin, scoparasin C, peniculascin I, peniculascin J, malformin E, fusicoccin A, peniprolin A, peniculascin K) with cytotoxic activity have been isolated from fungal entophytes [28, 29]. Compounds with cytotoxic effects isolated from endophytic fungi belong to various chemical groups such as aldehydes, alkaloids, chromones, benzofluoranthenes, cyclohexanones, depsidones, depsipeptides, ergochromes, esters, lignans, polyketides, spirobisnaphthalenes, diterpenes, sesquiterpenes, and xanthones. More than 100 anticancer compounds from endophytic fungi have been reported between 1990 and 2010. The cytotoxicity of these compounds against different cell lines (such as human acute monocytic leukemia cell line, A2780S ovarian tumor cell line, SW-620 colon tumor cell line, HCT-116 colon tumor cell line, MCF-7 breast cancer cell line, A549 lung cancer cell line, Vero cell line, U87MG and U138MG human glioblastoma cell lines) has been tested using the MTT assay and reported to exhibit high cytotoxic activity. The IC50 values of many reported anticancer compounds from endophytic fungi are similar to those of standard reference drugs (taxol, vincristine, vinblastine, and podophyllotoxin), indicating the potential of fungal endophytes in the development of anticancer drugs [30].

6.2 Antioxidant compounds

Antioxidants are known as oxidation inhibitors and are very active in combating reactive oxygen species (ROS). The discovery of new and healthy antioxidants from natural sources for fighting or preventing diseases is always essential. Secondary metabolites obtained from endophytic fungi (such as pestacin, isopestacin, 2,3,6,8-tetrahydroxy-1-methylxanthone, 5-(hydroxymethyl)-2-furanocarboxylic acid, rutin, cornicidin A and B, borineol, lapacol, coumarin, fluoroglusinol, and salidroside) can be potential sources of both known and new natural antioxidants [31–33]. These natural antioxidants may have anti-inflammatory, anti-tumor, antimutagenic, or anticancer activities. Antioxidants are considered the best chemical preventive agents against various human cancers. Antioxidant compounds from endophytic fungi are of great importance and can reduce the risk of diseases caused by oxidative damage [34].

6.3 Antimicrobial compounds

Endophytic fungi produce bioactive metabolites from their host plants to protect against various pathogens (bacteria, fungi, viruses, and protozoa). Compounds such as piperine, alterporriol A, 2-hydroxy-6-methyl benzoic acid, infumafungin, clavatulic acid, gestron, hydroxy gestron, pestacin, isopestacin, rutin, fumosorinone A, hypericin, 7-amino-4-methylcoumarin, zalarinone A, zalarinone B, zalaronic acid, clavatol, javanicin, verrucatol, fumosorithioamide A, pestalone, and fumosoripeptide have antimicrobial activity and have been isolated from fungal entophytes [35–37]. These antimicrobial compounds from endophytes have antibacterial, antifungal, antiviral, and antiprotozoal activities. Due to the increase in drug resistance in bacteria after long-term use of a known drug, researchers are always looking for new sources of antibiotics. Many endophytic fungi produce antibiotic compounds in a pure culture medium that have antibacterial activity against human and plant pathogenic bacteria. Natural compounds derived from endophytic fungi have high activity and lower toxicity compared to synthetic drugs [38].

6.4 Antiviral compounds

There is a global need for new antiviral compounds to address drug resistance issues. The inhibition of viruses by bioactive metabolites of endophytic fungi is significant. The potential discovery of antiviral compounds from endophytic fungi is in its early stages. The lack of suitable antiviral screening strategies in most compound discovery programs is a major limitation in the discovery of antiviral compounds from endophytic fungi. However, a few promising antiviral compounds, such as podophyllotoxin, S 39163/F-I, CR377, cytonic acid A and B, and cytosporone U from endophytic fungi have been reported. Antiviral compounds from endophytic fungi have been reported to exhibit activity against viruses such as human cytomegalovirus, influenza A virus (H1N1), and human immunodeficiency virus (HIV) [39–41].

6.5 Immune system suppressive compounds

Immune system suppressive drugs are used to prevent rejection of transplanted organs and maybe used to treat autoimmune diseases such as insulin-dependent diabetes and rheumatoid arthritis. Many immune system suppressive drugs are chemically ambiguous and heterogeneous in function, and their side effects can be challenging in long-term disease management. Since the discovery of cyclosporin A from *Trichoderma polysporum* (isolated from soil), this compound has been recognized as a major immune suppressive agent. However, this drug has serious side effects including kidney and nerve toxicity, infection risks, increased blood fat, and high blood pressure. Therefore, there is an urgent need to find effective and safe immune system suppressive drugs. Naturally occurring bioactive compounds from endophytic fungi such as sabineneol A and colutellin A may have great potential as safe immune system suppressive drugs for autoimmune diseases. These important compounds from endophytic fungi may fulfill a critical need for new immune suppressive drugs that could be beneficial for the treatment of autoimmune diseases and post-transplant care [28, 38, 42].

6.6 Antidiabetic compounds

Due to the side effects of alpha-glucosidase inhibitors (acarbose, voglibose, and miglitol), there is a need for new compounds with fewer side effects or no side effects. Compounds biosynthesized by endophytic fungi show strong antidiabetic activity and are cost-effective. Singh et al. isolated an endophytic fungus called *Cladosporium* sp. from *Tinospora cordifolia*, which exhibited strong inhibitory activity against alpha-glucosidase [43]. A bioactive compound called hydroxy-7,6-dimethoxy-3-methylisocoumarin obtained from the endophytic fungus Xylariaceae sp. isolated from the stem of *Quercus gilva* showed high inhibitory activity against alpha-glucosidase [44]. These studies indicate that endophytic fungi can be a potential source of antidiabetic compounds. **Table 1** shows the different activity of some bioactive compounds originating from endophytic fungi.

Compounds	Biological activity	Endophytic fungus	Host plant
Helvolic acid	Antibacterial	*Pichia guilliermondii*	*Paris polyphylla*
Pestalone	Antibacterial	*Chloridium* sp.	*Azadirachta indica*
Conidiogenone B	Antibacterial	*Penicillium chrysogenum*	*Laurencia* sp.
Khair acid	Antibacterial	*Curvularia papendorfii*	*Vernonia amygdalina*
Colletotric acid	Antibacterial	*Colletotrichum gloeosporioides*	*Artemisia mongolica*
Javanicin	Antibacterial	*Chloridium* sp.	*Azadirachta indica*
Brefeldin A	Anticancer	*Paecilomyces* sp.	*Torreya grandis*
Tauranin	Anticancer	*Phyllosticta spinarum*	*Platyclocarpus granatum*
Camptothecin	Anticancer	*Neurospora crassa*	*Camptotheca acuminata*
Beauvericin	Anticancer	*Fusarium oxysporium*	*Ephedra fasciculata*
Podophyllotoxin	Anticancer	*Trametes hirsuta*	*Podophyllum hexandrum*
Phomenone	Antifungal	*Xylaria* sp.	*Piper aduncum*
Mullein	Antifungal	*Pezicula livida*	*Fagus sylvatica*
Trichodermin	Antifungal	*Trichoderma harzianum*	*Ilex cornuta*
Flavipin	Antioxidant	*Chaetomium globosum*	*Ginkgo biloba*
Chlorogenic acid	Antioxidant	*Sordariomycete* sp.	*Eucommia ulmoides*
Corynesidones	Antioxidant	*Corynespora cassiicola*	*Lindenbergia philippensis*
Chaetopyranin	Antioxidant	*Chaetomium globosum*	*Polysiphonia urceolata*
Cytonic acids	Antiviral	*Cytonaema* sp.	*Quercus* sp.

Table 1.
Some compounds with antioxidant, antibacterial, antifungal, antiviral, and anticancer activities are obtained from endophyte fungi.

7. Challenges and perspectives in the study of endophytic fungi

Studying endophytic fungi is often challenging for researchers, as many endophytic fungi are not observed in plants, or they cannot be isolated and cultured, making it difficult. In addition, the methods used to study endophytes are incomplete, and better techniques are needed to better understand endophytic issues, including assessing the diversity and interactions of plant endophytes.

Lack of general awareness of the presence of endophyte communities in plant tissues has been a barrier to the advancement of the practical aspects of endophytes in agriculture. In the past, the common assumption that most plant endophytes are pathogenic has hindered a proper understanding of the role of endophytes in improving plant growth. In recent decades, a gradual development of research has shown that endophytes are common in plants and have a positive impact on plant growth and health, leading to significant progress in understanding the importance and function of endophytes. With the identification of the benefits of endophytic fungi for agriculture, companies producing bio-stimulants based on endophytic fungi have increased. To facilitate the development of microbial applications in agriculture, the recent United States Farm Bill of 2018 (also known as the Farm Bill 2018) in the United States and regulatory documents in the European Union explicitly address bio-stimulants and their regulations. It appears that a scientific, legal, and regulatory framework for some important future advancements in products and applications of endophytic microorganisms in agriculture will exist.

Conflict of interest

The authors declare no conflict of interest.

Author details

Mostafa Ebadi[1]* and Ali Ebadi[2]

1 Faculty of Basic Sciences, Department of Biology, Azerbaijan Shahid Madani University, Tabriz, Iran

2 Nuclear Agriculture Research School, Nuclear Science and Technology Research Institute, Karaj, Iran

*Address all correspondence to: ebadi2023@gmail.com

References

[1] Hyde K, Soytong K. The fungal endophyte dilemma. Fungal Diversity. 2008;**33**(163):163-173

[2] Krings M, Taylor TN, Hass H, Kerp H, Dotzler N, Hermsen EJ. Fungal endophytes in a 400-million-yr-old land plant: Infection pathways, spatial distribution, and host responses. New Phytologist. 2007;**174**(3):648-657. DOI: 10.1111/J.1469-8137.2007.02008.X

[3] Chareprasert S, Piapukiew J, Thienhirun S, Whalley AJS, Sihanonth P. Endophytic fungi of teak leaves *Tectona grandis* L. and rain tree leaves *Samanea saman* merr. World Journal of Microbiology and Biotechnology. 2006;**22**(5):481-486. DOI: 10.1007/S11274-005-9060-X/METRICS

[4] Rodriguez RJ, White JF, Arnold AE, Redman RS. Fungal endophytes: Diversity and functional roles. New Phytologist. 2009;**182**(2):314-330. DOI: 10.1111/J.1469-8137.2009.02773.X

[5] Dirzo R, Boege K. Patterns of herbivory and defense in tropical dry and rain forest. 2008. Available from: https://books.google.com/books/about/Tropical_Forest_Community_Ecology.html?id=ibsgvalaGOsC [Accessed: June 21, 2024]

[6] Schnitzer SA, Carson WP. Tropical forest community ecology. 2011. Available from: https://books.google.com/books?hl=en&lr=&id=ibsgvalaGOsC&oi=fnd&pg=PT11&dq=Hidden+Components+of+Tropical+Community+Ecology%3B+Schnitzer,+S.%3B+Carson,+W.,+Ed.%3B+Tropical+Forest+Community+Ecology&ots=Ligx_3G92X&sig=kgWZYzJCQ1pZ5auYIgfxAlp3ndI [Accessed: June 21, 2024]

[7] Bacon CW, Porter JK, Robbins JD, Luttrell ES. *Epichloe typhina* from toxic tall fescue grasses. Applied and Environmental Microbiology. 1977;**34**(5):576-581. DOI: 10.1128/AEM.34.5.576-581.1977

[8] Patterson CG, Potter DA, Fannin FF. Feeding deterrency of alkaloids from endophyte-infected grasses to Japanese beetle grubs. Entomologia Experimentalis et Applicata. 1991;**61**: 285-289. DOI: 10.1007/BF00187732

[9] Gentile A, Rossi MS, Cabral D, Craven KD, Schardl CL. Origin, divergence, and phylogeny of epichloë endophytes of native argentine grasses. Molecular Phylogenetics and Evolution. 2005;**35**(1):196-208. DOI: 10.1016/J.YMPEV.2005.01.008

[10] Kimmons CA, Gwinn KD, Bernard EC. Nematode reproduction on endophyte-infected and endophyte. Plant Disease. 1990;**74**(10):757-761

[11] Lee K. The effects of endophytic Fusarium Verticillioides on the interactions of maize and its fungal pathogen *Ustilago maydis*. 2010. Available from: https://conservancy.umn.edu/handle/11299/97147 [Accessed: June 21, 2024]

[12] Campanile G, Ruscelli A, Luisi N. Antagonistic activity of endophytic fungi towards *Diplodia corticola* assessed by in vitro and in planta tests. European Journal of Plant Pathology. 2007;**117**(3):237-246. DOI: 10.1007/S10658-006-9089-1/METRICS

[13] Tudzynski B, Sharon A. Biosynthesis, biological role and application of fungal phytohormones. Industrial Applications. 2002;**10**:183-211. DOI: 10.1007/978-3-662-10378-4_9

[14] Márquez LM, Redman RS, Rodriguez RJ, Roossinck MJ. A virus in a fungus in a plant: Three-way symbiosis required for thermal tolerance. Science. 2007;**315**(5811):513-515. DOI: 10.1126/SCIENCE.1136237/SUPPL_FILE/MARQUEZ-SOM-5811.PDF

[15] Orozco-Mosqueda MDC, Santoyo G. Plant-microbial endophytes interactions: Scrutinizing their beneficial mechanisms from genomic explorations. Current Plant Biology. 2021;**25**:100189. DOI: 10.1016/J.CPB.2020.100189

[16] Anyasi R, Atagana H. Endophyte: Understanding the microbes and its applications. Pakistan Journal of Biological Sciences. 2019;**22**(4):154-167

[17] Lu H, Wei T, Lou H, Shu X, Chen Q. A critical review on communication mechanism within plant-endophytic fungi interactions to cope with biotic and abiotic stresses. Journal of Fungi. 2021;**7**(9):719. DOI: 10.3390/JOF7090719

[18] Manias D, Verma A, Soni DK. Isolation and characterization of endophytes: Biochemical and molecular approach. Microbial Endophytes: Prospects for Sustainable Agriculture. 2020;**1**:1-14. DOI: 10.1016/B978-0-12-818734-0.00001-2

[19] Begerow D, Nilsson H, Unterseher M, Maier W. Current state and perspectives of fungal DNA barcoding and rapid identification procedures. Applied Microbiology and Biotechnology. 2010;**87**(1):99-108. DOI: 10.1007/S00253-010-2585-4/METRICS

[20] Cui J, Nie F, Zhao Y, Zhang D, Zhou D, Wu J, et al. A review on plant endophytes in response to abiotic stress. Environmental Pollutants and Bioavailability. 2024;**36**(1):1-17. DOI: 10.1080/26395940.2024.2323123

[21] de Carvalho JO, Broll V, Martinelli AHS, Lopes FC. Endophytic fungi: Positive association with plants. Molecular Aspects of Plant Beneficial Microbes in Agriculture. 2020;**2**:321-332. DOI: 10.1016/B978-0-12-818469-1.00026-2

[22] Tiwari P, Bae H. Trends in harnessing plant endophytic microbiome for heavy metal mitigation in plants: A perspective. Plants. 2023;**12**(7):1515. DOI: 10.3390/PLANTS12071515

[23] Qader MQ, Shekha YA. Role of environmental biotechnology in remediation of heavy metals by using fungal-microalgal strains. Basrah Journal of Agricultural Sciences. 2023;**36**(1):16-28. DOI: 10.37077/25200860.2023.36.1.02

[24] Eid AM, Salim SS, Hassan SED, Ismail MA, Fouda A. Role of endophytes in plant health and abiotic stress management. Microbiome in Plant Health and Disease: Challenges and Opportunities. 2019;**1**:119-144. DOI: 10.1007/978-981-13-8495-0_6

[25] Chaudhary P, Agri U, Chaudhary A, Kumar A, Kumar G. Endophytes and their potential in biotic stress management and crop production. Frontiers in Microbiology. 2022;**13**:933017. DOI: 10.3389/FMICB.2022.933017/BIBTEX

[26] Muthu Narayanan M, Ahmad N, Shivanand P, Metali F. The role of endophytes in combating fungal- and bacterial-induced stress in plants. Molecules. 2022;**27**(19):6549. DOI: 10.3390/MOLECULES27196549

[27] Gupta S, Chaturvedi P, Kulkarni MG, Van Staden J. A critical review on exploiting the pharmaceutical potential of plant endophytic fungi. Biotechnology Advances.

2020;**39**:107462. DOI: 10.1016/J.BIOTECHADV.2019.107462

[28] Ujam NT, Ajaghaku DL, Okoye FBC, Esimone CO. Antioxidant and immunosuppressive activities of extracts of endophytic fungi isolated from *Psidium guajava* and *Newbouldia laevis*. Phytomedicine Plus. 2021;**1**(2):100028. DOI: 10.1016/J.PHYPLU.2021.100028

[29] Prajapati J, Goswami D, Rawal RM. Endophytic fungi: A treasure trove of novel anticancer compounds. Current Research in Pharmacology and Drug Discovery. 2021;**2**:100050. DOI: 10.1016/J.CRPHAR.2021.100050

[30] Yin H, Zhou J, Lv H, Qin N, Chang FJ, Zhao X. Identification, pathogenicity, and fungicide sensitivity of ascochyta caulina (teleomorph: Neocamarosporium calvescens) associated with black stem on quinoa in China. Plant Disease. 2020;**104**(10):2585-2597. DOI: 10.1094/PDIS-09-19-2042-RE/ASSET/IMAGES/LARGE/PDIS-09-19-2042-RET4.JPEG

[31] Asomadu RO, Ezeorba TPC, Ezike TC, Uzoechina JO. Exploring the antioxidant potential of endophytic fungi: A review on methods for extraction and quantification of total antioxidant capacity (TAC). 3 Biotech. 2024;**14**(5):1-18. DOI: 10.1007/S13205-024-03970-3

[32] Gunasekaran S, Sundaramoorthy S, Anitha U, Sathiavelu M, Arunachalam S. Endophytic fungi with antioxidant activity-a review. Research Journal of Pharmacy and Technology. 2015;**8**(6):731-737. DOI: 10.5958/0974-360X.2015.00116.X

[33] Manganyi MC, Ateba CN. Untapped potentials of endophytic fungi: A review of novel bioactive compounds with biological applications. Microorganisms. 2020;**8**(12):1934. DOI: 10.3390/MICROORGANISMS8121934

[34] Mollaei S, Ebadi M. A review of phenolic antioxidants isolated from endophytic fungi. Journal of Plant Process and Function. 2022;**1**:99-117

[35] Silva DPD, Cardoso MS, Macedo AJ. Endophytic fungi as a source of antibacterial compounds—A focus on gram-negative bacteria. Antibiotics. 2022;**11**(11):1509. DOI: 10.3390/ANTIBIOTICS11111509

[36] Jha P, Kaur T, Chhabra I, Panja A, Paul S, Kumar V, et al. Endophytic fungi: Hidden treasure chest of antimicrobial metabolites interrelationship of endophytes and metabolites. Frontiers in Microbiology. 2023;**14**:1227830. DOI: 10.3389/FMICB.2023.1227830/BIBTEX

[37] Caruso DJ, Palombo EA, Moulton SE, Zaferanloo B. Exploring the promise of endophytic fungi: A review of novel antimicrobial compounds. Microorganisms. 2022;**10**(10):1990. DOI: 10.3390/MICROORGANISMS10101990

[38] Bourgaud F, Gravot A, Milesi S, Gontier E. Production of plant secondary metabolites: A historical perspective. Plant Science. 2001;**161**(5):839-851. DOI: 10.1016/S0168-9452(01)00490-3

[39] Adeleke BS, Babalola OO. Pharmacological potential of fungal endophytes associated with medicinal plants: A review. Journal of Fungi. 2021;**7**(2):147. DOI: 10.3390/JOF7020147

[40] Lacerda ÍC dos S, Polonio JC, Golias HC. Endophytic fungi as a source of antiviral compounds—A review. Chemistry and Biodiversity. 2022;**19**(6):e202100971. DOI: 10.1002/CBDV.202100971

[41] Nzimande B, Kumalo HM, Ndlovu SI, Mkhwanazi NP. Secondary metabolites produced by endophytic fungi, *Alternaria alternata*, as potential inhibitors of the human immunodeficiency virus. Frontiers in Genetics. 2022;**13**:1077159. DOI: 10.3389/FGENE.2022.1077159/BIBTEX

[42] Lin R, Kim H, Hong J, Li QJ. Biological evaluation of subglutinol a as a novel immunosuppressive agent for inflammation intervention. ACS Medicinal Chemistry Letters. 2014;**5**(5):485-490. DOI: 10.1021/ML4004809/SUPPL_FILE/ML4004809_SI_001.PDF

[43] Singh B, Kaur T, Kaur S, Manhas RK, Kaur A. An alpha-glucosidase inhibitor from an endophytic *Cladosporium* sp. with potential as a biocontrol agent. Applied Biochemistry and Biotechnology. 2015;**175**(4):2020-2034. DOI: 10.1007/S12010-014-1325-0/METRICS

[44] Indrianingsih AW, Tachibana S. α-Glucosidase inhibitor produced by an endophytic fungus, *Xylariaceae* sp. QGS 01 from *Quercus gilva* blume. Food Science and Human Wellness. 2017;**6**(2):88-95. DOI: 10.1016/J.FSHW.2017.05.001

Chapter 5

Exploring the Potential of *Serendipita indica* in Agriculture

Adolfo Posada, Rodrigo Patiño and Dagoberto Castro

Abstract

This document discusses the characteristics and applications of the facultative endophytic fungus *Serendipita indica*, emphasizing its colonization of plant roots, enhancement of nutrient absorption, and promotion of plant growth under stressful conditions. *S. indica* can grow axenically on synthetic growth media and its symbiotic association with various plant species is highlighted. The production of chlamydospores, which aid in plant resistance and survival, is described. Additionally, the document outlines methods for cultivating *S. indica*, including its propagation in liquid media and inoculation of in vitro *Mentha spicata* plantlets. Experimental results demonstrate the significant impact of *S. indica* on plant survival and biomass. Furthermore, the fungus's role in enhancing plant tolerance to pathogens and environmental stresses is discussed, highlighting its potential as a sustainable solution for improving plant development and agricultural productivity.

Keywords: endophytic root fungus, biotic stress, plant biostimulant, chlamydospores, *Mentha spicata*

1. Introduction

Serendipita indica is a facultative endophytic fungus belonging to the order Basidiomycetes. This fungus colonizes the roots of both monocotyledonous and dicotyledonous plants [1]. According to Varma et al. [2], *S. indica* shares many similarities with arbuscular mycorrhizal fungi (AMF), but unlike them, it can grow axenically in synthetic media. Colonization occurs in the root zone of plants and begins with the germination of chlamydospores, followed by the formation of a hyphal network in and within the root.

The hyphae branch out and continue to develop by penetrating the subepidermal layers of the root, with maximum colonization occurring in the zone of cellular differentiation [3]. Once the fungus is inside the plant, a symbiotic association develops.

Colonization by *S. indica* increases nutrient absorption, enabling plant survival under unfavorable abiotic conditions, such as drought, sudden temperature changes, and salinity stress. Additionally, it confers systemic resistance to toxins, heavy metal ions, and pathogenic organisms; it stimulates seed development and production [4, 5].

The mode of action of *S. indica* involves interactions with phytohormones, metabolites, photosynthates, and gene regulation. Assimilation of macronutrients, such as phosphorus, potassium, nitrogen, magnesium, and sulfur has been demonstrated in crops such as *Poncirus trifoliata*, *Triticum aestivum*, *Brassica napus*, *Oryza sativa*, *Panicum miliaceum*, and *Arabidopsis thaliana*, among others [6–8].

IntechOpen

S. indica promotes the production of various solutes in plants, such as proline, sucrose, polyols, glycine, and betaine, as well as antioxidant enzymes like catalase, ascorbate peroxidase, and superoxide dismutase, protecting various types of stress [9].

Similarly, colonization by *S. indica* in plant roots has been shown to enhance tolerance to bacterial pathogens, viruses, and fungal diseases. Some authors have demonstrated its action as a biocontrol agent against pathogens such as black spots in cabbage caused by *Alternaria brassicicola* [10], onion leaf blight caused by *Stemphylium* [11], and *Rhizoctonia solani* in tomato [12].

The purpose of this paper was to evaluate the production of the fungus *S. indica* in axenic nutrient media and to assess its effect on *M. spicata* plants inoculated under in vitro conditions.

2. Production of *S. indica* in synthetic culture media

The growth of this microorganism in synthetic culture media forms colonies that are white and velvety, with rapid radial growth. The mycelium is hyaline, with cylindrical hyphae having very thin walls typical of the fungus (**Figure 1A**). Spores in the shape of a pear, known as chlamydospores, are produced from these hyphae (**Figure 1B**).

2.1 Scale propagation of *S. indica* production

Commercial-scale propagation can be carried out in agitated liquid media at 110 rpm and 30°C (**Figure 2A**), and after 10–12 days, structures in the form of rounded cellular aggregates are formed (**Figure 2B**). Microscopic observations reveal mycelium and the beginning of chlamydospore formation (**Figure 2C**), and finally, spine-like structures form from which spores differentiate (**Figure 2D**). The concentration of chlamydospores was determined with the aid of a Neubauer chamber and was estimated at 1×10^6.

An important aspect is the production of chlamydospores, which correspond to enlarged vegetative cells with thick walls, exhibiting varied shapes and condensed cytoplasm, formed within hyphae or at the tips of hyphae. They have been observed in the three main clades of the fungal kingdom, particularly in the order of basidiomycetes [13].

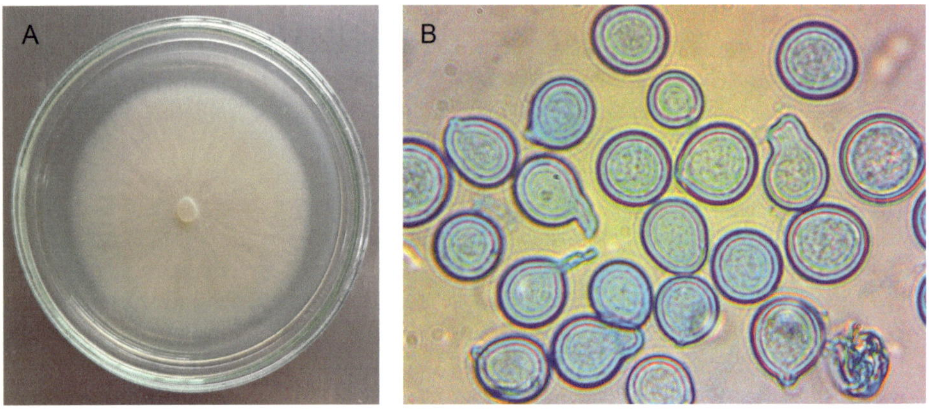

Figure 1.
Morphological characteristics of Serendipita indica. *A. Development of a colony of* S. indica *in a semisolid medium. B. Formation of chlamydospores in liquid media (photographs by Bioquirama S.A.S.).*

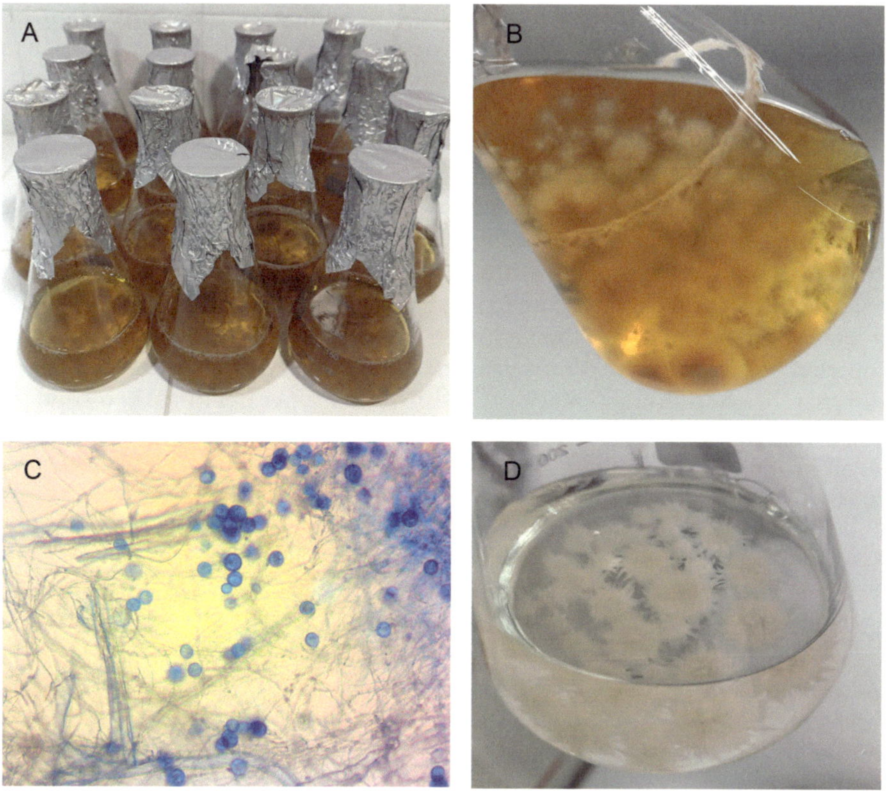

Figure 2.
Production scaling of Serendipita indica *in liquid media. A. Cultivation of* S. indica *mycelium in liquid medium under agitation. B. Formation of cellular aggregates of mycelium. C. Microscopic observation of the mycelium. D. Formation of spine-like structures. (Photographs by Bioquirama S.A.S.).*

Among the biological functions of chlamydospores, their resistance to dehydration stands out. They are produced within plant roots during drought and are transported in fragments. They germinate when they encounter favorable conditions of moisture and temperature.

2.2 Plant material

Microplants shoots of *Mentha spicata* were developed in an MS medium [14], supplemented with 3% sucrose and 0.5 mg/L benzyladenine in a semisolid medium, and were used as source materials. Rooting of plantlets was conducted under completely aseptic conditions in a culture medium composed of MS mineral salts added with 3% sucrose, 0.5 mg/L indole butyric acid, and 0.7% agar-agar. The internodes were planted in nine plastic boxes, each containing 15 plantlets, and incubated at 28°C with a photoperiod of 12 hours light, using fluorescent light lamps FFF 80 $\mu mol\ m^{-2}\ s^{-1}$. Thirty days after sowing, plantlets formed roots.

2.3 In vitro inoculation of *S. indica* in *Mentha spicata* shoots

The inoculum was prepared from a suspension of *S. indica* spores in sterile water in 2-mL microtubes. Spore concentration was determined using a Neubauer chamber.

Inoculations with the microorganisms consisted of adding a suspension of 2 mL of *S. indica* to the in vitro plantlets under aseptic conditions at a final concentration of 1.0×10^5 spores/mL.

2.4 Evaluation of the effect of microplants biotization on survival during the acclimatization phase and dry biomass

Using the aforementioned methodology, in vitro rooted plantlets were inoculated with *S. indica* and left to incubate for 10 days (**Figure 3A**). Then microplants were transferred to a humid chamber and planted in seedling trays with peat moss, previously sterilized with autoclave for 3 hours at 121°C (**Figure 3B**). The plants were kept for a period of 30 days, after which measurements of survival and growth of the seedlings were made. A randomized trial with 45 plants per treatment was conducted, where the treatments corresponded to plants biotized with *S. indica* and a control group of plantlets without endophyte. For the determination of dry mass, five plants were randomly selected from each treatment. The entire plants were weighed on an analytical balance (MF) and then placed in an oven with a forced draft of air at 65°C until constant weight.

2.5 Assessment of survival and dry mass of hardened *M. spicata* seedlings

According to the results shown in **Figure 4A**, significant differences were observed regarding the survival of seedlings during the acclimatization process. Seedlings inoculated with *S. indica* exhibited a 90.5% survival rate, whereas control plants had a 76% survival rate. Similarly, the dry mass of plants inoculated with *S. indica* averaged 0.55 g/plant, while control plants averaged 0.37 g/plant (**Figure 4B**).

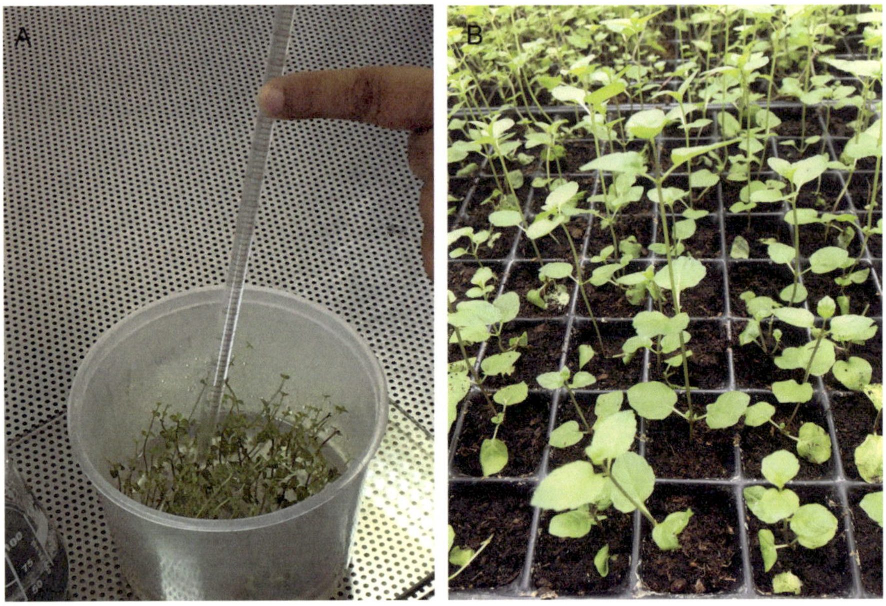

Figure 3.
Inoculation and acclimatization process of M. spicata *plants. A. In vitro inoculation of plants during the rooting phase with* S. indica *fungus. B. Acclimatization of plants produced in vitro in seed trays.*

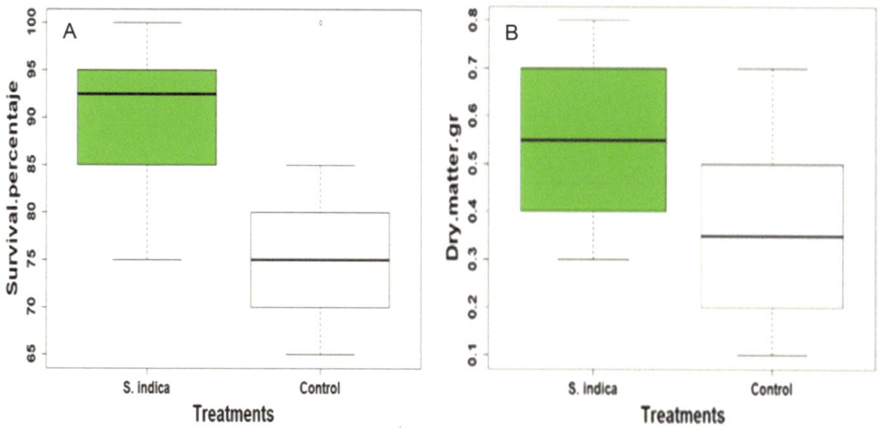

Figure 4.
Response of Mentha spicata *plants to in vitro inoculation with* Serendipita indica*. A. Percentage of survival of* M. spicata *seedlings. B. Dry biomass of 30-day-old seedlings. Significant differences were found between the means of the treatments (P < 0.05; Tukey HSD).*

Ref. [15] Indicated that *S. indica* is a microorganism that assists plants in growth, nutrient absorption, and environmental stress tolerance when in coexistence with them. Inoculated plants respond positively to *S. indica* through various mechanisms, including improved root development and plant growth, which may explain the results obtained with *M. spicata* [16]. Additionally, it enhances water and nutrient absorption [17].

The results obtained from the symbiosis of *S. indica* with *M. spicata* included an increase in dry mass, which, according to Nanda et al. [18], this fungus aids in enhancing chlorophyll contents and photosynthetic rates, thereby improving plant development.

2.6 Determination of root colonization of *M. spicata* by *S. indica*

Thirty days after transplanting to seedling germination trays, root samples were taken, and staining was performed according to the techniques described by Phillip and Hayman [19]. Roots were washed with water and cut into 1.0 cm fragments, then placed in a 10% KOH solution for 15 minutes. Subsequently, root segments were neutralized with 1 N HCl and thoroughly washed with water. Staining was conducted with a 0.05% trypan blue solution for 12 hours and then mounted in lactophenol for microscopic observations. Fragments were placed in a hemocytometer for analysis under a microscope. Colonization was evaluated using the method of Giovannetti and Mose [20]. The percentage of colonization was calculated as follows:

$$\text{Percentage of Colonization} = \begin{pmatrix} \text{Number of Colonized Segments /} \\ \text{Total Number of Observed Segments} \end{pmatrix}^{*} 100 \quad (1)$$

2.7 Colonization by *S. indica*

According to the results shown in **Table 1**, the colonization percentage was 70%.

Microscopic studies of *M. spicata* roots treated with *S. indica* revealed extensive inter- and intracellular root colonization with chlamydospores (**Figure 5A** and **B**). Hifal colonization was observed on the root surface and in the intercellular and intracellular spaces of the root cortex. Chlamydospores were found in both single

Treatment	Colonization percentage (%)
Plants inoculated with *S. indica*	70
Control (non-inoculated plants)	0

Table 1.
Colonization of S. indica *in* M. spicata *roots.*

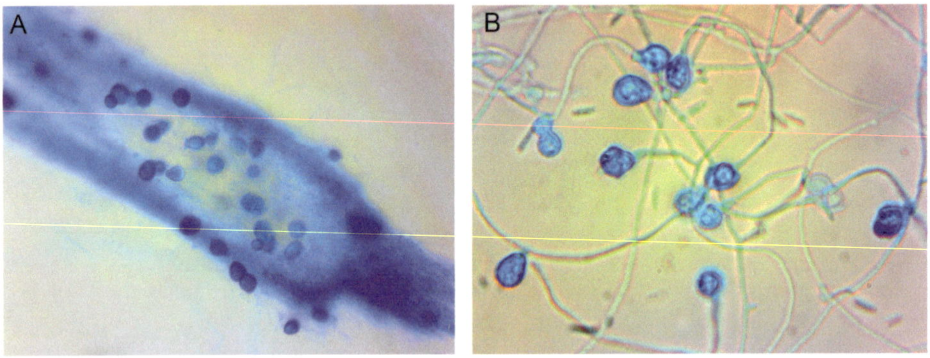

Figure 5.
Spores of S. indica *were observed under a conventional microscope. A. Root of* M. spicata *with inter- and intracellular spores. B. Spores in areas adjacent to the root zone.*

and double spore forms. The spore shapes varied from round to ovoid, with some exhibiting the typical pear-shaped structure.

3. Conclusions

The endophytic fungus *S. indica* can be cultivated on a large scale in liquid culture media at concentrations of 1.0×10^6 spores/mL, making it a viable option for enhancing plant development. One advantage is that chlamydospores are produced, which serve as resistance structures that associate with roots, positively impacting plant development and physiology.

Inoculating *M. spicata* seedlings under in vitro conditions with *S. indica* revealed its endophytic nature, with a 70% root colonization rate. Plants treated with the endophyte exhibited a survival rate of 90.5% and a higher percentage of dry biomass, which correlates with improved plant development.

S. indica shows promise as an endophytic microorganism, providing plants with protection against both biotic and abiotic stresses by regulating various processes. These include the synthesis of antioxidant substances, osmolytes, secondary metabolites, and phytohormones related to defense mechanisms. Consequently, it plays a crucial role in enhancing global food security by positively influencing plant development, production, and quality. As a result, it presents itself as an environmentally sustainable and economically viable solution.

Acknowledgements

The authors are especially grateful to BIOQUIRAMA S.A.S and Universidad Católica de Oriente (UCO) for their contribution to the development of this study.

Conflict of interest

The authors declare no conflict of interest.

Author details

Adolfo Posada[1], Rodrigo Patiño[1] and Dagoberto Castro[2]*

1 Bioquirama S.A.S. Antioquia, Colombia

2 Universidad Católica de Oriente, Rionegro, Colombia

*Address all correspondence to: dcastro@uco.edu.co

References

[1] Osman M, Stigloher C, Mueller M, Waller F. An improved growth medium for enhanced inoculum production of the plant growth-promoting fungus *Serendipita indica*. Plant Methods. 2020;**2020**(16):39

[2] Varma A, Sherameti I, Prasad R, Das A, Sharma A, et al. Symbiotic fungus *Piriformospora indica*: Review. In: Hock B, editor. The Mycota IX. Fungal Associations. 2nd ed. Berlin Heidelberg: Springer-Verlag; 2012. pp. 231-254

[3] Saleem S, Sekara A, Pokluda R. *Serendipita indica*—A review from agricultural point of view. Plants. 2022;**11**:3417

[4] Varma A, Savita V, Sudha J, Sahay N, Butehorn B, Franken P. *Piriformospora indica,* a cultivable plant-growth-promoting root endophyte. Applied and Environmental Microbiology. 1999;**5**(6):2741-2744

[5] Harman GE. Multifunctional fungal plant symbiont: New tools to enhance plant growth and productivity. The New Phytologist. 2011;**189**:647-649

[6] Yang L, Zou YN, Tian ZH, Wu QS, Kuča K. E effects of beneficial endophytic fungal inoculants on plant growth and nutrient absorption of trifoliate orange seedlings. Scientia Horticulturae. 2021;**277**:109815

[7] Bakhshandeh E, Pirdashti H, Lendeh KS, Zahra G, Khanghahi MY, Crecchio C. Effects of plant growth promoting microorganisms inoculums on mineral nutrition, growth and productivity of rice (*Oryza sativa L.*). Journal of Plant Nutrition. 2020;**43**:1643-1660

[8] Su ZZ, Wang T, Shrivastava N, Chen YY, Liu X, Sun C, et al. Piriformospora indica promotes growth, seed yield and quality of *Brassica napus L*. Microbiological Research. 2017;**199**:29-39

[9] Hayat S, Hayat Q, Alyemeni MN, Wani AS, Pichtel J, Ahmad A. Role of proline under changing environments: A review. Plant Signaling and Behavior. 2012;**7**:1456-1466

[10] Saleem S, Bytešníková Z, Richtera L, Pokluda R. The effects of *Serendipita indica* and guanidine-modified nanomaterial on growth and development of cabbage seedlings and black spot infestation. Agriculture. 2021;**11**:1295

[11] Roylawar P, Khandagale K, Randive P, Shinde B, Murumkar C, Ade A, et al. Piriformospora indica primes onion response against Stemphylium leaf blight disease. Pathogens. 2021;**10**:1085

[12] Del Barrio-Duque A, Ley J, Samad A, Antonielli L, Sessitsch A, Compant S. Beneficial endophytic bacteria-*Serendipita indica* interaction for crop enhancement and resistance to phytopathogens. Frontiers in Microbiology. 2019;**10**:2888

[13] Kues U. Life history and developmental processes in the basidiomycete *Coprinus cinereus*. Microbiology and Molecular Biology Reviews. 2000;**64**:316-353

[14] Murashige T, Skoog FA. Revised medium for rapid growth and bioassays with tobacco tissue culture. Physiologia Plantarum. 1962;**15**:473-497

[15] Ghorbani A, Razavi S, Omran VG, Pirdashti H. *Piriformospora indica* alleviates salinity by boosting redox poise and antioxidative potential of tomato. Russian Journal of Plant Physiology. 2018;**65**:898-907

[16] Hosseini F, Mosaddeghi MR, Dexter AR, Sepehri M. Effect of endophytic fungus *Piriformospora indica* and PEG-induced water stress on maximum root growth pressure and elongation rate of maize. Plant and Soil. 2019;**435**:423-436

[17] Padash A, Shahabivand S, Behtash F, Aghaee A. A practicable method for zinc enrichment in lettuce leaves by the endophyte fungus *Piriformospora indica* under increasing zinc supply. Scientia Horticulturae. 2016;**213**:367-372

[18] Nanda R, Agrawal V. *Piriformospora indica*, an excellent system for heavy metal sequestration and amelioration of oxidative stress and DNA damage in Cassia angustifolia Vahl under copper stress. Ecotoxicology and Environmental Safety. 2018;**156**:409-419

[19] Phillip JM, Hayman DS. Improved procedures for clearing roots and staining parasitic and VAM fungi for rapid assessment of infection. Transactions of the British Mycological Society. 1970;**55**:158-116

[20] Giovannetti M, Mosse B. An evaluation of techniques for measuring vesicular-arbuscular mycorrhizal infection in roots. New Phytologist. 1980;**84**:489-500

Section 3

Fungal Pathogenesis

Chapter 6

Near-Infrared Hyperspectral Imaging and Thermal Imaging Techniques for Rapid Diagnosis of Anthracnose in Mango Pre- and Post-Harvest

Panmanas Sirisomboon, Cheewanun Dachoupakan Sirisomboon, Panan Rerngsamran and Sneha Sharma

Abstract

The advent of machine vision systems and the emergence of specialized sensors like multispectral, hyperspectral and thermal cameras have brought about a technological transformation in various industries, particularly in autonomously conducting quality checks on pre- and post-harvested agriculture including fungus detection in laboratories, on tree and canopy images. NIR spectral region has a better ability to identify the defects than the visible range images since the NIR region can present absorption bands of a large variation of molecular information consisting of biochemical and physiochemical information of fruits. This technique is more suitable for disease detection. The detection of disease in damaged fruit due to fungal infection was possible due to the change in temperature within the region of interest in the thermal images, while the UAV-borne infrared camera suggested a small temperature increase with a pathogen increase. NIR-HSI and thermal imaging provide promising results for the rapid detection of pathogens in fruits, enhancing food safety measures.

Keywords: fruits, fungal infection, computer vision, early detection, non-destructive techniques

1. Introduction

Thailand is best known for its variety of exotic fruits and serves the best flavors in the world. A recent survey showed that Thailand exported approximately 93 million USD worth of fresh mangoes in a single year. The data from the Department of Agriculture, Thailand, investigated that the most common storage problem for mangoes was the harmful residues and flies in the skin of mangoes causing post-harvest spoilage. Several plant diseases can significantly affect the quality of fruits. Some examples can be potato leaf disease, black rust fungus in wheat, coffee rust, powdery mildew in grasses, vegetables, shrubs, and trees, and anthracnose in mangoes, vegetables, and trees [1]. The advent of machine vision systems and the emergence of specialized sensors like multispectral and hyperspectral cameras have brought about a technological transformation in various industries, particularly agribusiness. This shift is attributed to the utilization of vision systems capable of autonomously conducting quality checks on pre- and post-harvested agri-food products. Several literatures have reported that hyperspectral imaging has shown potential for inspecting, characterizing and controlling tools for agricultural and horticultural products [2–5].

The quality of mango has been estimated based on internal parameters such as titratable acidity (TA), firmness, total soluble solids (TSS), and dry matter contents. The internal quality index and ripening index (RPI) are some other important indicators for quality monitoring. An application of a handheld NIR spectrometer was studied for identifying the TSS and pH of mango by Lamptey et al. [6]. The authors applied several preprocessing techniques with multivariate classification models using support vector machine (SVM), linear discriminant analysis (LDA), neural network (NN), and random forest (RF). The study shows that non-destructive assessment has the potential to assess the TSS and pH of mango using handheld NIR integrated with chemometric tools [6].

Particularly, tropical fruit crops are vulnerable to infection by *Colletotrichum* species, which is commonly known as anthracnose [7]. **Figure 1** shows the cycle of how the anthracnose disease occurs, in which phase, and how it develops in the fruits [7].

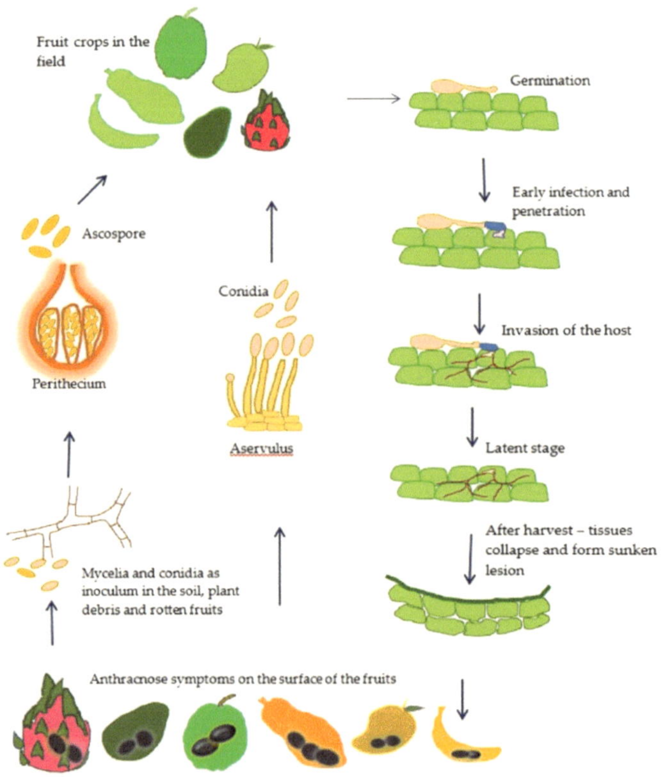

Figure 1.
Anthracnose disease cycle of tropical fruit crops (adapted from [7]).

The reason for post-harvest diseases in these fruits is due to the infection and development of anthracnose pathogens in an inactive or latent stage [7]. Anthracnose pathogens not only affect fruits but also target other parts of plants, such as leaves, flowers, twigs, and branches. The conidia or spores produced within these infected tissues are then liberated and spread during rainy days through water splashes or during periods of high humidity [8]. Consequently, these serve as the main source of inoculation for fruit infection during the pre-harvest stage [8].

2. Hyperspectral imaging (HSI) for anthracnose detection

Anthracnose poses a significant threat to mango crops in major production areas, impacting approximately 60% of the yield [9]. However, hyperspectral imaging technology offers a non-invasive approach to the early detection and assessment of internal damage, presenting a promising solution [9]. HSI is an advanced optical technology that can detect agricultural products' internal and external information including fungal infections and diseases. The hypercube created from the HSI image includes both spatial and spectral data, enabling the construction of a spatial map that highlights spectral differences [10]. Research into the NIR-HSI technique holds significant promise for automatic target detection and for analyzing the composition of various substances [11].

Velásquez et al. [12] develop a system for detecting anthracnose in mango fruits using Vis–NIR hyperspectral imaging and discriminant analysis. The HSI system used for imaging each fruit comprised a hemispherical dome with 12 halogen lamps, a monochromatic camera (Photometrics CoolSnap ES) with sensitivity from 320 to 1030 nm, and two liquid crystal tunable filters (LCTF). The filters operated in the visible (450–720 nm) (Varispec VIS07) and near-infrared (730–980 nm) (Varispec NIR07) ranges, as illustrated in **Figure 2** [12].

Velásquez et al. [12] aimed to investigate the feasibility of early anthracnose detection in two mango cultivars using hyperspectral imaging and machine learning techniques. Their research uncovered potential correlations between various feature wavelengths and anthracnose, resulting in developing a robust model for spectral anthracnose detection in mangoes. Mangoes were inoculated with *Colletotrichum*

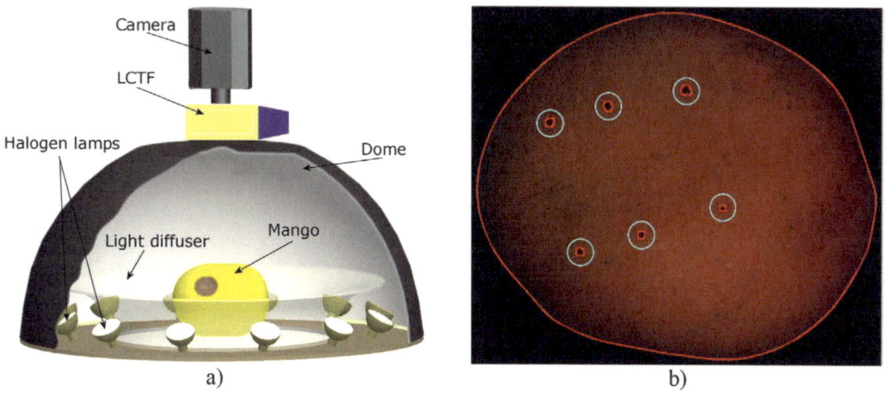

Figure 2.
Vis–NIR hyperspectral imaging system for image acquisition. (a) Region of interest (ROI) of the mango sample (b) (Adapted from Velásquez et al., [12]).

gloeosporioides spores, and hyperspectral images of both control and infected fruit were captured in the 450–970 nm spectral range. Additionally, another application of a push-scan hyperspectral imaging system (Model HSI-VNIR-0001, Shanghai Wuling Optoelectronics Technology Co., Ltd., Shanghai, China) featuring a spectral camera, light source, dark box, and computer with a spectral range of 373–1033 nm was employed to identify and differentiate early-stage anthracnose in strawberries [13].

3. Thermal imaging (TI) for anthracnose detection

The thermal imaging (TI) system comprises infrared (IR) detectors, signal-processing components, and image acquisition modules. These detectors absorb IR energy emitted by objects, converting it into electrical signals. Subsequently, the signal processing unit translates these signals into thermal images.

There are some works reported for the early detection of fungal infection and anthracnose disease in fruits and vegetables using thermal image processing. With an advancement in computer vision, the detection of crop diseases through the extraction of red, green, and blue (RGB) images is made possible. Zhu et al. [14] identified tomato mosaic disease and white leaf rust using infrared thermal images in the early stages. Naik and Patel [15] developed a classification method to estimate the state of maturity of the Langdo mango, from thermal images with a mean intensity algorithm in L*a*b* color space and FLIR ONE thermal camera is used to predict the maturity of the mango. The accuracy to grade mango in 2.3 seconds was achieved by approximately 89% [15].

A case study was done by Mahanti et al. [16] to detect the bruise in apples using a TI camera. The bruise was created manually at room temperature and kept at the average temperature of 25°C for 30 minutes. The result showed that the average temperature of fresh tissue (29°C) was lower than the bruised tissue as shown in **Figure 3**. In another study conducted by Lipińska et al. [17], the growth of *Penicillium expansum*, *Botrytis cinerea*, and *Rhizopus stolonifer* on apples infected with these fungi was examined through temperature measurements taken with a thermovision

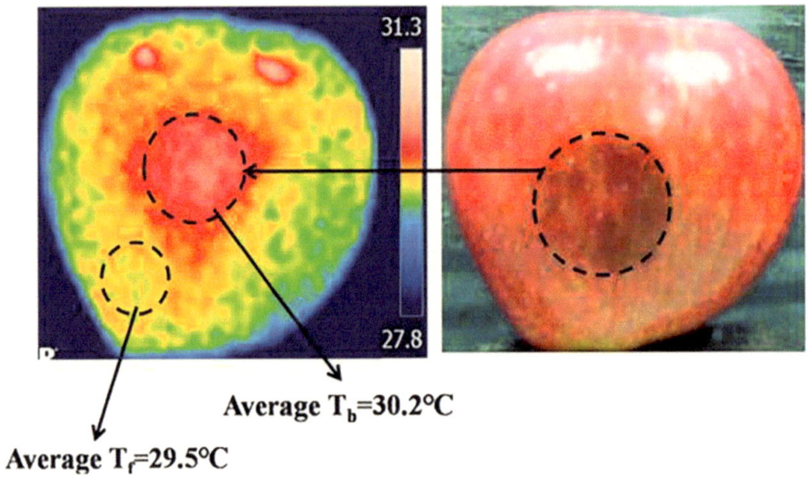

Figure 3.
Thermal image of bruised apple [16].

camera. The results revealed a significant relationship between the temperature of the apples and the growth of the microbes, demonstrating a clear two-stage temperature pattern. Initially, there was an increase in temperature observed in contaminated apples on the first day, followed by a subsequent decrease.

Additionally, the feasibility of using an infrared thermal camera to classify the fungal-infected wheat grains was studied by [18]. The classification model attained the maximum accuracy of 100% to identify the healthy and unhealthy grains based on the thermal images [18].

The study examined various diseases affecting guava, including anthracnose, algal spot, fruit flies, and style end rot, using local binary pattern (LBP) and principal component analysis (PCA) techniques for extracting features and reducing dimensionality [19, 20]. The results showed that the detection of disease in damaged guava due to fungal infection was possible due to the change in temperature within the region of interest in the thermal images of guava [19]. The accuracy of fruit quality prediction was higher than 99% using CNN architecture trained on dehydrated and diseased guava [19].

Infrared thermographic was applied to detect the leaf moisture and physiological stress condition of Japanese spindle (*Euonymus japonica* Thunb.) and glossy pivot (*Ligustrum sinense)* in a low-temperature environment [21]. The results demonstrated that thermography could effectively detect scorched leaf areas, twig dieback, and the sap warming phenomenon in leaves [21].

Jiao et al. [22] presented a novel approach for assessing pesticide drift in real-time, utilizing infrared thermal imaging technology to detect temperature variations pre- and post-spraying. Subsequently, they quantified the dispersion and concentration distribution of droplets. The infrared thermal imaging system, in conjunction with image processing algorithms, was employed to detect drift distribution and spray coverage. Ground and aerial spray applications were both investigated in the experiment resulting in the efficacy of the thermal imaging to detect the temperature differences during spray application.

4. Detection of pathogen including anthracnose by on tree fruit image and canopy image

Crop ground imaging is the technique of acquiring a crop's fruit and leave image at ground level using smartphone and digital cameras. Several researchers incorporated this technique to acquire the image of fruit and tree leaves in field conditions. Multispectral imaging (MSI) and HSI have indicated their ability to detect crop disease in different growth stages. HSI was employed to identify anthracnose diseases in tea plants, achieving a detection accuracy of 98% at the leaf level and 94% at the pixel level [23]. They have also identified the specific wavelengths that are disease-sensitive at bands 542, 686 and 754 nm [23]. Using computer vision, a database with images taken on a tree's healthy, diseased, and plagued blueberry leaves was collected by Sulla et al. [24] to develop image processing and compare the performance of machine learning algorithms for classification. The method attained the healthy and diseased classification accuracy of 84% using deep learning. Jin et al. [25] utilized the HSI-visible NIR system to acquire an image of field wheat *Fusarium* head blight disease. The experimental setup is shown in the **Figure 4**. The model's test results indicate that the two-dimensional convolutional bidirectional gated recurrent unit neural network (2D-CNN-BidGRU) achieved an F1 score of 0.750 and an accuracy of 0.743.

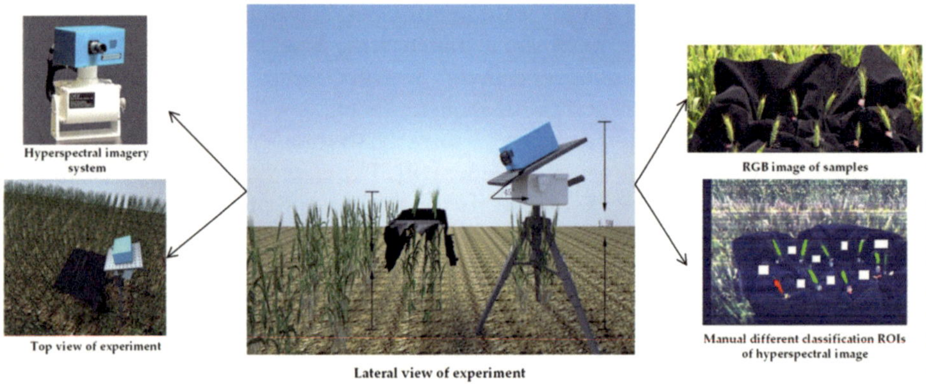

Figure 4.
Hyperspectral image acquisition of wheat with blight disease setup at field level [26].

Alaa et al. [26] developed a mobile application with the real-time detection of common diseases mentioned before by mobile cameras and also Red Palm Weevil by acquiring thermal images of palm trees using thermal cameras connected to smartphones. The image processing and enhancement were done before developing the CNN and SVM models for classification. The CNN and SVM models attained an accuracy of 97.9 and 92.8%, respectively [26].

Smigaj et al., [27] investigated the use of a low-cost fixing-wing UAV-borne thermal system for monitoring disease-induced canopy temperature rise. At the canopy level, the comparison of tree crown temperature recorded by the UAV-borne infrared camera suggested a small temperature increase with a pathogen increase with a correlation of 0.527.

4.1 Pathogen detection using NIR-HSI and thermal image

Non-destructive methods such as NIR spectroscopy, mid-IR spectroscopy, and nuclear magnetic resonance (NMR) have been aggressively used to detect pathogens and fungal infections in fruits. NIR spectroscopy is an advanced technique to predict the quality traits, defects, and textural parameters of the fruits. As spectroscopic techniques only obtain the information of a point, it does not enable simultaneous acquisition of spectra from different regions of fruits at the same time. Hyperspectral imaging also known as imaging spectrographs compensates for these drawbacks of spectroscopy by integrating imaging and spectral information of the sample with different data acquisition modes. Jiang et al. [28] conducted a study to compare the ability of different HSI systems at visible and short near-infrared regions to detect post-harvest disease in winter jujubes. The result indicated that the vis–NIR spectral region has a better ability to identify the post-harvest defects in fruit. Since the vis–NIR region can present absorption bands of a large variation of molecular information consisting of biochemical and physiochemical information of fruits, this technique is more suitable for disease detection [29].

The mean reflectance Vis–NIR and SWIR spectra of jujubes from the HSI system are shown in **Figure 5** in two control groups and black spot disease inoculated jujubes at six infection periods [29]. The mean spectra of the infected spectra showed a downward trend in the vis–NIR and SWIR region during the 5-day storage [29]. It was explained additional opportunities were given for light to interact with the cellular

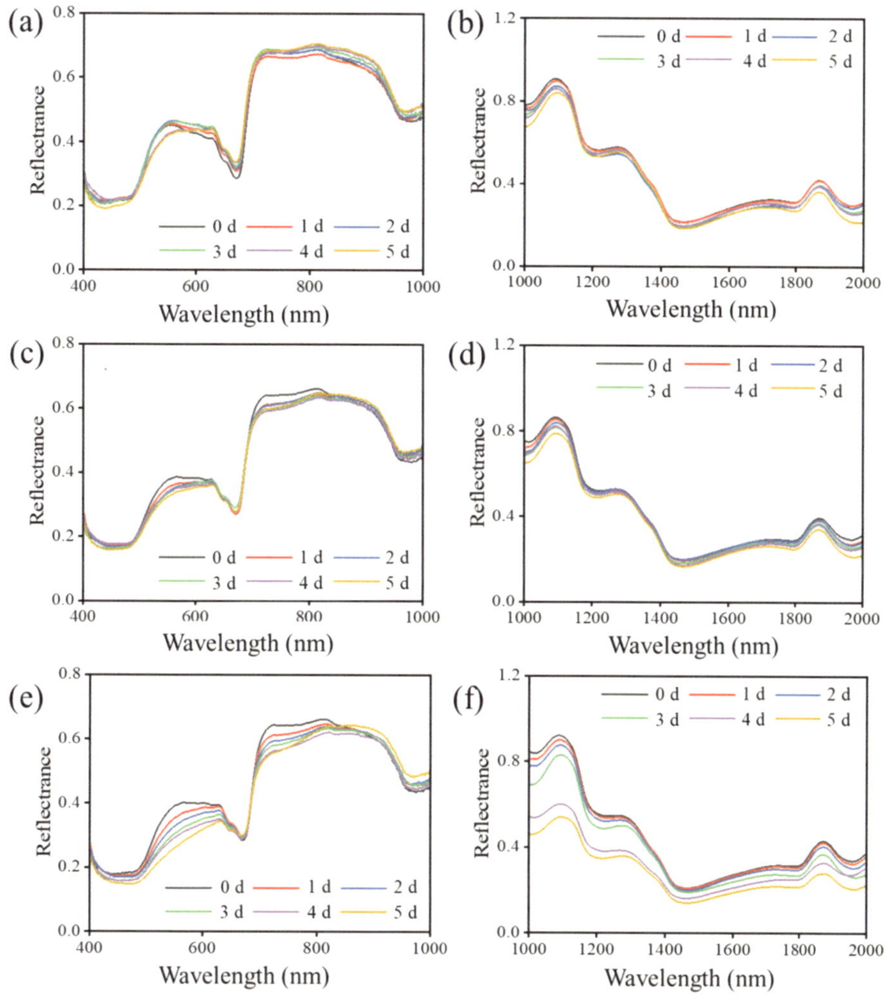

Figure 5.
Comparison of mean spectra from control and infected groups during the storage at 20° C in the vis–NIR (400–1000) and SWIR (1000–2000 nm) region mean spectra of (a) healthy sample without treatment (control group I) in vis–NIR region, (b) control group I in SWIR region, (c) control group in II in vis–NIR region, (d) control group II in SWIR region, (e) infected group of sample in Vis–NIR, and (f) infected sample in SWIR [29].

matter, leading to increased absorption and scattering as the cellular structure of the flesh tissue underwent progressive damage [29]. The result showed that HSI had the potential for the detection of black spot disease on winter jujubes and showcased that the implication of this technique for the disease detection and disease process visualization on fruits is more accurate and convenient.

Another example shows the efficacy of the HSI system for assessing strawberry foliar anthracnose [30]. This study shows the feasibility of using the HSI system and identifies important wavelengths for healthy and unhealthy strawberry leaf classification [30]. The average spectral signature for each infection stage from the three experiments is presented in **Figure 6**. It was identified that it was visually possible to distinguish healthy and unhealthy samples, but it was not easy to classify the spectra by observing the spectra for infection stages. Using multivariate techniques, different infection stages were distinguishable [30].

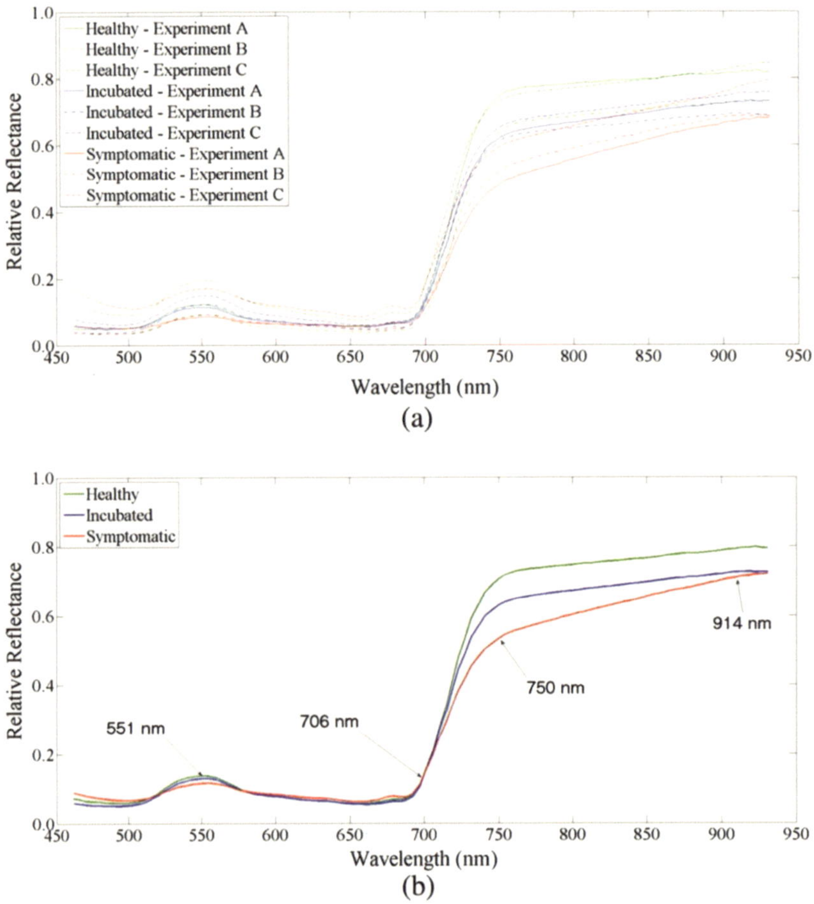

Figure 6.
Mean spectral signature for each strawberry anthracnose infection stage: (a) different experiments, and (b) with optimal wavelengths [30].

Siripatrawan and Makino [31] applied HSI integrated with machine learning for rapid identification of quiescent infection of anthracnose in mango fruit. In this study, a non-destructive approach was developed to diagnose the pre-symptomatic anthracnose infection on mango fruit and classify the level of the symptom's development. The HSI yielded spectral patterns that could be employed to identify and describe anthracnose symptoms associated with both the metabolic by products and the deteriorated fruit tissues resulting from fungal invasion [31].

Infrared thermal imaging can potentially detect pathogens in fruits because pathogens often induce changes in the physiological and biochemical properties of infected fruits, which can lead to alterations in their thermal profiles. This technique relies on the detection of differences in temperature distribution across the surface of the fruit, which can be indicative of underlying physiological changes caused by pathogens. Thermal imaging provides a non-invasive and promising method for identifying pests and diseases in fruits by utilizing the unique thermal signatures of infected or infested produce, which stem from changes in their metabolic activity.

Stoll et al. [32] performed an experiment using thermal imagery to determine the sensitivity of the temperature change for pathogen detection in grapevines under different water stress conditions. The result indicated that, with irrigated vines, pathogen development caused an increase in leaf temperature and vines under water stress showed lower temperature at the sites. The result suggested that early and remote detection using thermal imagery has the potential for pre-symptomatic diagnosis of biotic stress [32].

Infrared thermography elucidated the fluctuation in temperature of infected apple leaves when studying scab disease [33]. They discovered that the maximum temperature difference (MTD) rose as scabs developed, closely linked to the size of infection sites. However, in advanced stages, MTD declined due to leaf aging, while leaf transpiration increased throughout the scab development stages. Consequently, MTD not only distinguishes diseased from healthy leaves but also aids in disease quantification.

5. Conclusion

HSI and thermal imaging provide promising results for the rapid detection of pathogens in fruits, enhancing food safety measures. HSI capture spectral and spatial information from a wide range of wavelengths, allowing for detailed analysis of the surface characteristics of fruits. This technique enables the detection of subtle changes associated with the presence of pathogens, such as alterations in color, texture, and biochemical composition. By analyzing healthy and infected fruits' images and spectral information, HSI systems can effectively differentiate between them, facilitating early detection and mitigation of pathogen contamination.

Additionally, thermal imaging provides valuable insights into the physiological responses of fruits to viral and bacterial pathogens. The infected fruits exhibit more altered metabolic activities, leading to variations in temperature distribution across their surfaces. Thermal imaging cameras detect these temperature discrepancies, enabling the identification of potential hotspots indicating the presence of pathogens. Integrating machine learning and deep learning algorithms with thermal imaging and HSI further enhances anthracnose or other pathogen detection accuracy by combining important surface morphology and physiological data. These non-destructive imaging techniques offer a rapid and comprehensive approach to screening fruits for pathogen contamination, thereby minimizing the risk of foodborne illnesses.

Author details

Panmanas Sirisomboon[1], Cheewanun Dachoupakan Sirisomboon[2], Panan Rerngsamran[2] and Sneha Sharma[3]*

1 Department of Agricultural Engineering, School of Engineering, King Mongkut's Institute of Technology, Ladkrabang, Bangkok, Thailand

2 Faculty of Science, Department of Microbiology, Chulalongkorn University, Bangkok, Thailand

3 Department of Infrastructure Engineering, The University of Melbourne, Victoria, Australia

*Address all correspondence to: sharmasneha0725@gmail.com

References

[1] Wongsila S, Chantrasri P, Sureephong P. Machine learning algorithm development for detection of mango infected by anthracnose disease. In: *2021 Joint International Conference on Digital Arts, Media and Technology with ECTI Northern Section Conference on Electrical, Electronics, Computer and Telecommunication Engineering*. Cha-am, Thailand: IEEE; 2021. pp. 249-252

[2] Velásquez C, Prieto F, Palou L, Cubero S, Blasco J, Aleixos N. New model for the automatic detection of anthracnose in mango fruits based on Vis/NIR hyperspectral imaging and discriminant analysis. Journal of Food Measurement and Characterization. 2024;**18**(1):560-570. DOI: 10.1007/s11694-023-02173-3

[3] Rungpichayapichet P, Mahayothee B, Nagle M, Khuwijitjaru P, Müller J. Robust NIRS models for non-destructive prediction of postharvest fruit ripeness and quality in mango. Postharvest Biology and Technology. 2016;**111**:31-40. DOI: 10.1016/J.POSTHARVBIO.2015.07.006

[4] dos Santos Neto JP, de Assis MWD, Casagrande IP, Cunha Júnior LC, de Almeida Teixeira GH. Determination of 'palmer' mango maturity indices using portable near infrared (VIS-NIR) spectrometer. Postharvest Biology and Technology. 2017;**130**:75-80. DOI: 10.1016/J.POSTHARVBIO.2017.03.009

[5] Sharma S et al. Near-infrared hyperspectral imaging combined with machine learning for physicochemical-based quality evaluation of durian pulp. Postharvest Biology and Technology. 2023;**200**:112334. DOI: 10.1016/J.POSTHARVBIO.2023.112334

[6] Lamptey FP, Teye E, Abano EE, Amuah CLY. Application of handheld NIR spectrometer for simultaneous identification and quantification of quality parameters in intact mango fruits. Smart Agricultural Technology. 2023;**6**:100357. DOI: 10.1016/J.ATECH.2023.100357

[7] Zakaria L. Diversity of Colletotrichum species associated with anthracnose disease in tropical fruit crops—A review. Agriculture. 2021;**11**(4):297. DOI: 10.3390/AGRICULTURE11040297

[8] Fitzell RD, Peak CM. The epidemiology of anthracnose disease of mango: Inoculum sources, spore production and dispersal. Annals of Applied Biology. 1984;**104**(1):53-59. DOI: 10.1111/J.1744-7348.1984.TB05586.X

[9] Velásquez C, Prieto F, Palou L, Cubero S, Blasco J, Aleixos N. New model for the automatic detection of anthracnose in mango fruits based on Vis/NIR hyperspectral imaging and discriminant analysis. Journal of Food Measurement and Characterization. 2024;**18**(1):560-570. DOI: 10.1007/S11694-023-02173-3/TABLES/7

[10] Sharma S, Sumesh KC, Sirisomboon P. Rapid ripening stage classification and dry matter prediction of durian pulp using a pushbroom near infrared hyperspectral imaging system. Measurement. 2021;**189**:110464. DOI: 10.1016/j.measurement.2021.110464

[11] ElMasry G, Sun DW. Principles of hyperspectral imaging technology. Hyperspectral Imaging for Food Quality Analysis and Control. Academic Press. 2010:3-43. DOI: 10.1016/B978-0-12-374753-2.10001-2

[12] Velásquez C, Aleixos N, Gomez-Sanchis J, Cubero S, Prieto F, Blasco J. Enhancing anthracnose detection in mango at early stages using hyperspectral imaging and machine learning. Postharvest Biology and Technology. 2024;**209**:112732. DOI: 10.1016/J.POSTHARVBIO.2023.112732

[13] Liu C, Cao Y, Wu E, Yang R, Xu H, Qiao Y. A discriminative model for early detection of anthracnose in strawberry plants based on hyperspectral imaging technology. Remote Sensing. 2023;**15**(18):4640. DOI: 10.3390/RS15184640

[14] Zhu W, Chen H, Ciechanowska I, Spaner D. Application of infrared thermal imaging for the rapid diagnosis of crop disease. IFAC-PapersOnLine. 2018;**51**(17):424-430. DOI: 10.1016/J.IFACOL.2018.08.184

[15] Naik S, Patel B. Thermal imaging with fuzzy classifier for maturity and size based non-destructive mango (Mangifera Indica L.) grading. In: *2017 International Conference on Emerging Trends and Innovation in ICT, ICEI 2017*. Pune, India: IEEE; 3-5 Feb 2017. pp. 15-20. DOI: 10.1109/ETIICT.2017.7977003

[16] Mahanti NK et al. Emerging non-destructive imaging techniques for fruit damage detection: Image processing and analysis. Trends in Food Science and Technology. 2022;**120**:418-438. DOI: 10.1016/J.TIFS.2021.12.021

[17] Lipińska E, Pobiega K, Piwowarek K, Błażejak S. Research on the use of thermal imaging as a method for detecting fungal growth in apples. Horticulturae. 2022;**8**(10):972. DOI: 10.3390/HORTICULTURAE8100972

[18] Chelladurai V, Jayas DS, White NDG. Thermal imaging for detecting fungal infection in stored wheat. Journal of Stored Products Research. 2010;**46**(3):174-179. DOI: 10.1016/J.JSPR.2010.04.002

[19] Pathmanaban P, Gnanavel BK, Anandan SS. Guava fruit (Psidium guajava) damage and disease detection using deep convolutional neural networks and thermal imaging. The Imaging Science Journal. 2022;**70**(2):102-116. DOI: 10.1080/13682199.2022.2163536

[20] Almutiry O et al. A Novel Framework for Multi-Classification of Guava Disease. DOI: 10.32604/cmc.2021.017702

[21] Wang F, Omasa K, Xing S, Dong Y. Thermographic analysis of leaf water and energy information of Japanese spindle and glossy privet trees in low temperature environment. Ecological Informatics. 2013;**16**:35-40. DOI: 10.1016/J.ECOINF.2013.04.006

[22] Jiao L, Dong D, Feng H, Zhao X, Chen L. Monitoring spray drift in aerial spray application based on infrared thermal imaging technology. Computers and Electronics in Agriculture. 2016;**121**:135-140. DOI: 10.1016/J.COMPAG.2015.12.006

[23] Yuan L et al. Detection of anthracnose in tea plants based on hyperspectral imaging. Computers and Electronics in Agriculture. 2019;**167**:105039. DOI: 10.1016/J.COMPAG.2019.105039

[24] Sulla C, Molina C, Rodriguez C, Fernandez T. Diseases detection in blueberry leaves using computer vision and machine learning techniques. International Journal of Machine Learning and Computing. 2019. Available from: https://www.ijmlc.org/vol9/854-A006.pdf;**9**(5):656-661 Accessed: May 03, 2024

[25] Jin X, Jie L, Wang S, Qi HJ, Li SW. Classifying wheat hyperspectral pixels of healthy heads and fusarium head blight disease using a deep neural network in the wild field. Remote Sensing. 2018;**10**(3):395. DOI: 10.3390/RS10030395

[26] Alaa H, Waleed K, Samir M, Tarek M, Sobeah H, Salam MA. An intelligent approach for detecting palm trees diseases using image processing and machine learning. IJACSA International Journal of Advanced Computer Science and Applications. 2020;**11**(7):434-441. Available from: www.ijacsa.thesai.org [Accessed: May 03, 2024]

[27] Smigaj M, Gaulton R, Barr SL, Suárez JC. UAV-borne thermal imaging for forest health monitoring: Detection of disease-induced canopy temperature increase. The International Archives of the Photogrammetry, Remote Sensing and Spatial Information Sciences. 2015;**XL-3-W3**(3W3):349-354. DOI: 10.5194/ISPRSARCHIVES-XL-3-W3-349-2015

[28] Jiang M et al. Study on Black Spot Disease Detection and Pathogenic Process Visualization on Winter Jujubes Using Hyperspectral Imaging System. 2023. DOI: 10.3390/foods12030435

[29] Liu G et al. Application of near-infrared hyperspectral imaging for detection of external insect infestations on jujube fruit. International Journal of Food Properties. 2016;**19**(1):41-52. DOI: 10.1080/10942912.2014.923439

[30] Yeh YH, Chung WC, Liao JY, Chung CL, Kuo YF, Te Lin T. Strawberry foliar anthracnose assessment by hyperspectral imaging. Computers and Electronics in Agriculture. 2016;**122**:1-9. DOI: 10.1016/J.COMPAG.2016.01.012

[31] Siripatrawan U, Makino Y. Hyperspectral imaging coupled with machine learning for classification of anthracnose infection on mango fruit. Spectrochimica Acta. Part A, Molecular and Biomolecular Spectroscopy. 2024;**309**:123825. DOI: 10.1016/J.SAA.2023.123825

[32] Stoll M, Schultz HR, Berkelmann-Loehnertz B. Exploring the sensitivity of thermal imaging for Plasmopara viticola pathogen detection in grapevines under different water status. Functional Plant Biology. 2008;**35**(4):281-288. DOI: 10.1071/FP07204

[33] Oerke EC, Fröhling P, Steiner U. Thermographic assessment of scab disease on apple leaves. Precision Agriculture. 2011;**12**(5):699-715. DOI: 10.1007/S11119-010-9212-3/TABLES/2

Chapter 7

The Xiangya Lesion: A Paradigm Shift in Understanding Fungal Pathogenesis

Xiujuan Yan and Charles Xiaoxiang Zhu

Abstract

This chapter presents a comprehensive examination of the Xiangya Lesion, a novel entity resulting from the interaction between the fungus Aspergillus sydowii and human keratinocytes within plantar hyperkeratosis-like lesions. The discovery of these "zombie cells," formed by integrating the fungus with the host's cellular machinery, profoundly impacts our understanding of fungal pathogenesis, treatment modalities, and the broader evolutionary strategies of fungi within the human host. The pathogen's intracellular nature may render traditional antifungal agents ineffective, necessitating the development of novel diagnostic techniques and therapeutic strategies to manage this condition effectively. Through an interdisciplinary exploration of the Xiangya Lesion, this chapter aims to shed light on the complex world of fungal infections and contribute to the ongoing battle between pathogen and host.

Keywords: Xiangya Lesion, Aspergillus sydowii, fungal pathogenesis, persistence and recurrence of fungal infections, resistance to antifungal drugs, intracellular fungal infection

1. Introduction

The fungal world, a realm of astonishing diversity, harbors both beneficial and harmful species. While some fungi play vital roles in ecosystems and human health, others cause devastating diseases [1, 2]. Understanding how fungi interact with their hosts is crucial for developing effective treatments and preventing outbreaks. This chapter explores a groundbreaking discovery that challenges our understanding of fungal pathogenesis: the "Xiangya Lesion."

Based on research by Zhu et al., the Xiangya Lesion represents a unique manifestation of fungal infection characterized by the formation of "zombie cells"—human keratinocytes hijacked and manipulated by fungal cells [3]. This novel finding, observed in plantar hyperkeratosis-like lesions, suggests a previously unknown complexity in fungal-host interactions. This chapter explores the implications of this discovery, highlighting its potential to shift our understanding of fungal pathogenesis and the development of new therapeutic strategies.

This chapter will address the following:

- The discovery and characterization of the Xiangya Lesion.
- The unique features of "zombie cells" and their implications for fungal pathogenesis.
- The potential of the Xiangya Lesion as a model system for studying fungal-host interactions.
- The implications of this discovery for developing new antifungal therapies.

By exploring the Xiangya Lesion, this chapter aims to illuminate the intricate and often surprising ways fungi interact with their hosts, paving the way for a deeper understanding of fungal pathogenesis and the development of more effective treatments.

2. The discovery of zombie cells

The discovery of zombie cells has been revolutionary in medical mycology. These composite entities, resulting from the union of Aspergillus sydowii and human keratinocytes, have challenged long-held paradigms of fungal pathogenesis. This section delves into the intricate details of this discovery, from the initial observations that led to the hypothesis to the rigorous scientific process that confirmed the existence of these enigmatic cells.

The story begins with the persistent puzzle of plantar hyperkeratosis, a condition often attributed to mechanical stress and other noninfectious factors [4, 5]. However, some lesions displayed characteristics that did not align with the conventional understanding of the disease. The meticulous examination of these lesions led to the first hints of an unconventional pathogen at play [6, 7].

Researchers, led by Charles Xiaoxiang Zhu, hypothesized that an unidentified pathogen might contribute to forming hyperkeratotic lesions [3]. This hypothesis stemmed from the observation that these lesions often coincided with fungal infections, were notoriously difficult to cure, and had high relapse rates. The team investigated this possibility using histological examinations, cell culture techniques, and genetic sequencing.

The serendipitous discovery of zombie cells emerged from a meticulous investigation into plantar hyperkeratosis-like lesions (**Figures 1** and **2**). These lesions, typically appearing as thickened skin on the soles of the feet, were found to harbor more than just the usual suspects of fungal infections. Groundbreaking research led by Charles Xiaoxiang Zhu unveiled a novel phenomenon: Aspergillus sydowii forming composite cells with human keratinocytes, termed "zombie cells." [3].

Initial observations and hypothesis formation: Histological evaluation of the lesions using H&E, PAS, and immunochemistry revealed the unexpected presence of anucleated squamous cells containing basophilic bodies. This peculiar finding led researchers to hypothesize the involvement of an unconventional pathogen, prompting the exploration of Aspergillus sydowii as a potential culprit (**Figure 3**).

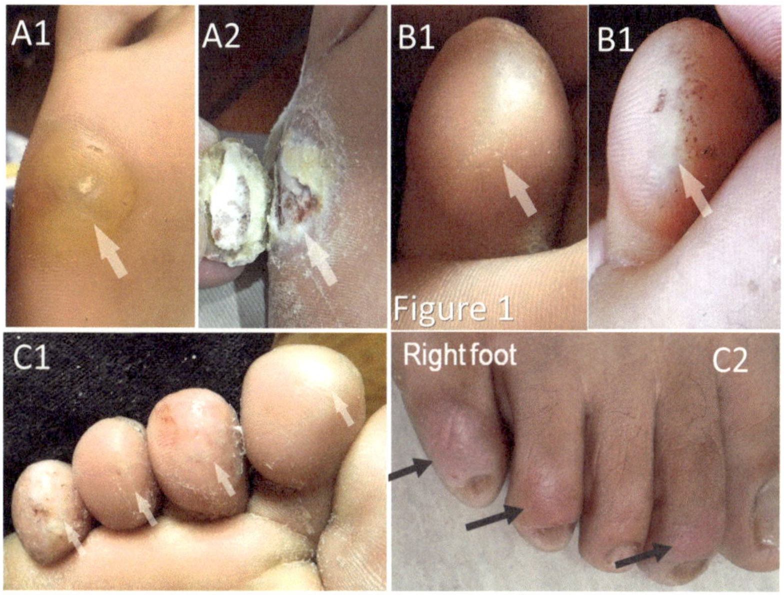

Figure 1.
Xiangya Lesions on right foot. A: A Xiangya Lesion manifested as a plantar callus, measuring 28 × 30 mm² (A1). After partial trimming, the lesion was treated with 100 mg of aspirin powder to soften the hyperkeratotic tissue, resulting in a white appearance, and with 100 mg of terbinafine or itraconazole powder to inhibit fungal growth, which led to pigmented dark gray and brown colors. B: A hyperkeratotic growth on the small toe, with B2 showing fungal growth on the lesion during humid, rainy weather in early autumn. C1: Softened Xiangya Lesions on the toes resembling tinea pedis in rainy weather. C2: Dermatitis-like Xiangya Lesion on the dorsal aspect of the toes and onychomycosis-like nail Xiangya Lesions.

Cultural revelations and zombie cells: Culturing infected skin tissue in ATG293, a human cell culture medium designed to support the growth of both human skin tissue and fungal pathogens, led to a remarkable observation. Within days, hyphae growth was observed, and over weeks, a tumor-like mass emerged (**Figure 2C**). This mass, composed exclusively of epithelial cells, underwent a transformation, eventually giving rise to fungal balls, indicating the presence of viable fungal elements within the anucleated epithelial cells (**Figure 2D, F, W, X**) [3].

Genetic sequencing and pathogen identification: Aspergillus sydowii was confirmed as the causative agent through genetic sequencing. Fungal genomic DNA extracted from the cultured cells was amplified using PCR targeting the ribosomal RNA gene. Comparing the obtained DNA sequences to known fungal genomes led to the identification of Aspergillus sydowii (**Figure 2T**).

Characteristics of zombie cells: Transmission electron microscopy (TEM) revealed distinct features of the zombie cells. They lacked human nuclei and contained numerous inclusion bodies (approximately 0.4–0.7 μm in diameter) surrounded by abundant rough endoplasmic reticulum (RER) and polyribosomes, indicative of active divisions (**Figure 4**). These inclusion bodies were morphologically consistent with fungal nuclei, suggesting a unique form of intracellular survival for the fungus.

Implications of the discovery: The discovery of zombie cells has profound implications for our understanding of fungal infections. It suggests that certain fungi have

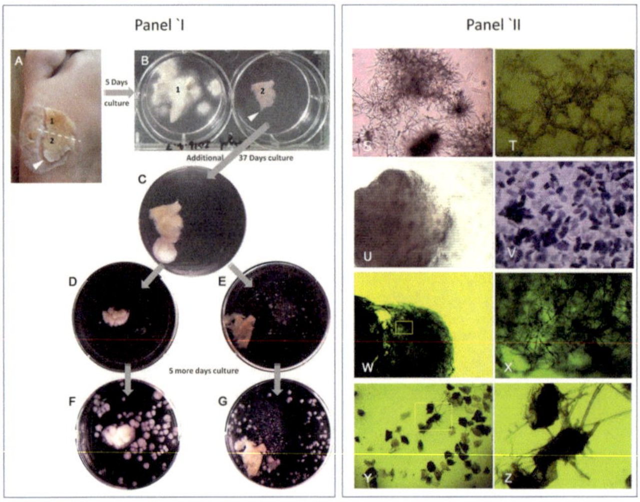

Figure 2.
Discovery of intracellular fungal infection of skin keratinocytes. Panel I (Xiangya Lesion culture in human cell culture media): A) Hyperkeratotic tissue was trimmed from the plantar lesion and divided into two pieces. B) The tissue pieces were placed in the wells of a 6-well culture plate with 2.5 ml of ATG293 medium and incubated at 37°C for 5 days. Multiple molds were observed in culture B1, while budding growth for the tissue was seen in culture B2, as indicated by the white arrows. C) After five additional weeks of incubation at 37°C, a tumor-like mass measuring 9 × 8 × 7.5 mm^3 grew out from the lesion tissue. D, F) The tumor-like tissue was broken up, and the pieces were further incubated in a fresh culture medium. E, G) The non-tumor portion of the lesion tissue was also incubated with fresh medium, and after 5 days. Panel II (microscopic photos corresponding to Panel I): T) Fungus photographed in a liquid culture, corresponding to Figure B1. U, V) The fresh tumor-like tissue from Figure D was examined directly under a microscope or after staining with trypan blue for 15 minutes, revealing that the tumor was composed of keratinocytes of variable sizes, approximately 20–40 μm in length. W, X) Microscopic photos corresponding to the culture of Figure F, in which the tumor-like tissue resulted in the disappearance of the tumor cells and the replacement by fungal balls. Y, Z) The culture of Figure G was stained with trypan blue and examined under a microscope, showing fungal hyphae growing and breaking out from the epithelial cells.

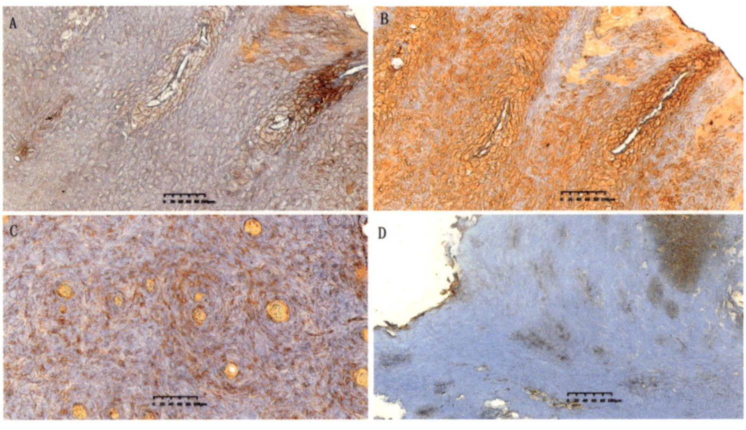

Figure 3.
Immunohistochemical findings. A, B: Microscopic images of consecutive tissue sections of the hyperkeratotic lesion on the right fifth toe with positive immunohistochemical staining using anti-epithelial membrane antigen (EMA) antibodies (A) and anti-Aspergillus soluble proteins (ASP) antibodies (B). C, D: Microscopic images of the positive staining of the plantar callus-like lesion (C) and of the negative staining of a hand callus (D), respectively, stained with anti-ASP antibodies.

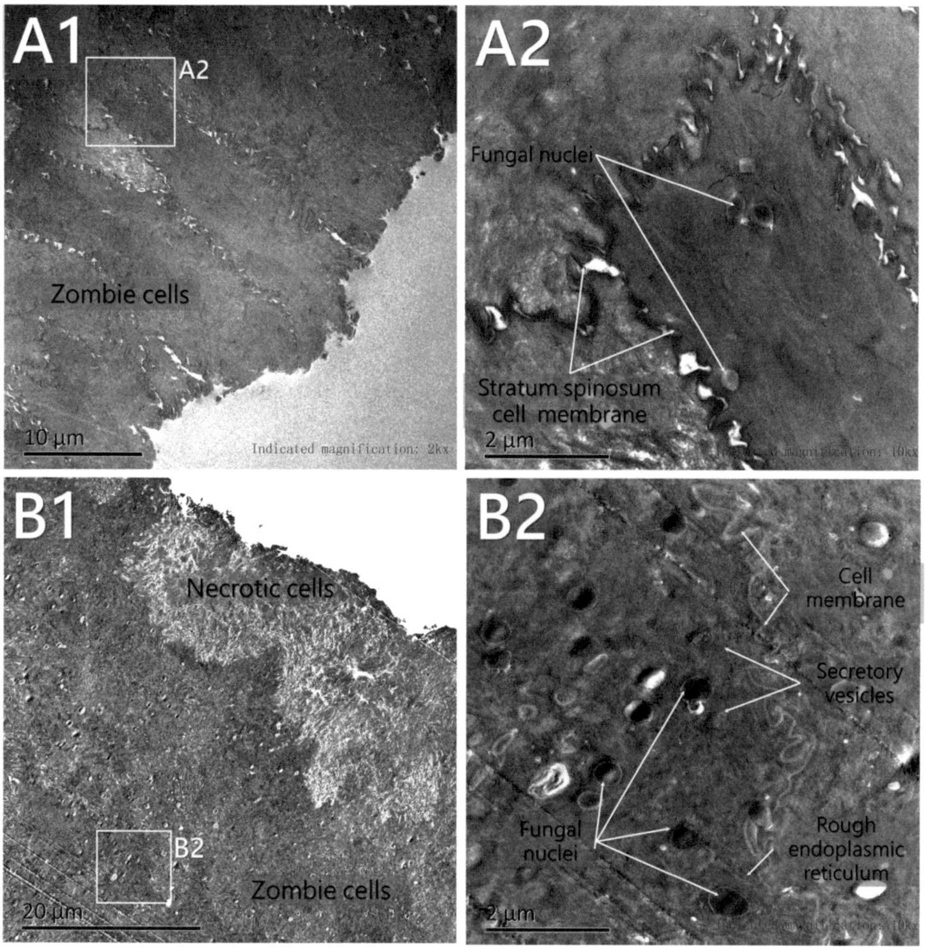

Figure 4.
Electronic microscopic examinations of Xiangya Lesions. TEM images from biopsies of the right plantar (A) and fifth toe (B) hyperkeratotic lesions showed stratum spinosum cells, some of which were irregular shapes and sizes. All cells lacked human nuclei, and some cellular membranes had filament-filled cytoplasmic spines and desmosome structures. Many inclusion bodies approximately 0.4–0.7 um in diameter was observed in the cytoplasm of the cells, surrounded by abundant rough endoplasmic reticulum (RER) and polyribosomes, some of which exhibited active divisions. A1 and B1: Irregular epithelial cells of the right foot plantar callus-like lesion and the right small toe hyperkeratotic lesion, respectively. A2 and B2: Focal magnifications of A1 and B1, respectively, to observe the subcellular structures and fungal nuclei.

evolved to integrate with human cells, potentially evading the host's immune response and conventional antifungal treatments. This finding necessitates a reevaluation of treatment strategies for fungal infections, focusing on developing new therapeutic approaches that can target the intracellular forms of these pathogens [6].

3. Formation mechanisms of composite cells: a detailed exploration

The development of composite cells, or "zombie cells," within plantar hyperkeratosis-like lesions presents a biological enigma that challenges our understanding of cellular biology and pathogenesis. This section delves into the potential formation mechanisms of these unique entities, considering the biological processes that may lead to the fusion of fungal and human cells.

3.1 Initial infection and internalization

The formation of composite cells is believed to begin with Aspergillus sydowii entering the host tissue, potentially through microlesions or natural skin openings like hair follicles and sweat glands. The fungus may secrete enzymes that degrade the extracellular matrix, facilitating its penetration into the epidermis [8].

3.2 Intracellular survival and evasion of host defenses

Once internalized, Aspergillus sydowii must evade the host's immune response to survive intracellularly. The fungus is theorized to manipulate the host cell's machinery, possibly by suppressing apoptosis, modulating signaling pathways, or exploiting the host's nutrient supply to create a survival-conducive niche [9, 10].

3.3 Formation of anucleated epithelial cells and integration of fungal elements

Observations of anucleated epithelial cells within hyperkeratotic lesions suggest a process where the host cell's nucleus is either expelled or degraded, creating a cellular structure suitable for fungal integration. The subsequent integration of fungal elements with these cells may involve endocytosis-like mechanisms, leading to the formation of composite cells [11].

3.4 Development of nucleus-like bodies and proliferation

The composite cells exhibit nucleus-like bodies that stain positively for fungal proteins, indicating a form of modified fungal nuclei within the host cell. These cells can proliferate, contributing to lesion overgrowth (**Figure 2**), potentially due to the interference of fungal components with the host cell's growth regulatory mechanisms [12].

3.5 Transformation, disease recurrence, and pathogenesis implications

Environmental or cellular changes may trigger the composite cells' ability to revert to natural fungal forms, leading to tissue destruction and infection spread, which may explain disease recurrence. This capacity has significant implications for fungal pathogenesis, offering an explanation for the chronicity and treatment resistance observed in plantar hyperkeratosis [13].

3.6 Future research directions and conclusion

Elucidating the molecular interactions during composite cell formation is vital for developing therapeutic strategies. Future research should identify the factors and pathways involved in this process and determine the genetic changes within the host cell. The formation of composite cells in plantar hyperkeratosis-like lesions is a complex interaction between the human host and the fungal pathogen, and further research is essential for advancing our understanding and treatment of these infections [14].

4. Implications for fungal pathogenesis

The identification of composite cells, or "zombie cells," within plantar hyperkeratosis-like lesions has profound implications for our understanding of fungal pathogenesis. This novel form of fungal infection may significantly alter our approach to diagnosing, treating, and preventing fungal diseases.

4.1 Redefining fungal-host interactions

The traditional view of fungal infections involves the invasion of host tissues by extracellular fungal elements, which are then targeted by the immune system and medical interventions [15]. However, the existence of zombie cells suggests a more nuanced interaction where the fungus and host cells merge. This allows the pathogen to potentially evade immune detection and therapeutic efforts [3].

4.2 Challenges in detection and diagnosis

The ability of *Aspergillus sydowii* to form composite cells presents a significant challenge for the detection and diagnosis of fungal infections. Standard mycological examinations may fail to identify the pathogen hidden within host cells. This necessitates developing new diagnostic techniques to detect fungal genetic material or proteins within host cells [2].

4.3 Resistance to antifungal therapies

The formation of composite cells may contribute to the resistance of certain fungal infections to antifungal treatments. Many antifungal drugs target the fungal cell wall or membrane, which may be ineffective if the fungus is shielded within the host cell [16]. This resistance mechanism could explain the high relapse rates and difficulty in curing some fungal infections [17].

4.4 Evolutionary adaptations of fungi

The formation of composite cells could represent an evolutionary adaptation that allows fungi to survive in a hostile host environment. By integrating with host cells, fungi may gain access to nutrients and a protective niche while avoiding immune surveillance. Understanding this adaptation can provide insights into the evolutionary pressures that drive pathogenicity in fungi [18–20].

4.5 Impact on host immune response

The presence of composite cells may alter the host's immune response to fungal infections. The immune system may recognize the composite cells as foreign, leading to inflammation and tissue damage. Conversely, it may be deceived into tolerating the fungal presence, allowing the infection to persist [21, 22].

4.6 Role in chronic infections and recurrences

The formation of composite cells may play a critical role in the chronicity of certain fungal infections and their tendency to recur. These cells can transform back into infectious fungal forms, which could be a key factor in the relapse of symptoms after treatment. Understanding this transformation process could reveal new targets for preventing recurrence [23, 24].

4.7 Broader implications for mycology

The discovery of zombie cells has broader implications for mycology. It raises questions about the prevalence of similar composite cells in other fungal infections and suggests that fungi may have a greater capacity for intracellular survival than previously recognized. This could lead to a reevaluation of existing fungal disease models and the development of new research directions [25].

4.8 Development of novel therapeutic strategies

The implications of composite cell formation for fungal pathogenesis necessitate developing novel therapeutic strategies. These may include drugs that can penetrate host cells to target intracellular fungi, immunomodulatory therapies that enhance the host's ability to clear infected cells and genetic approaches that disrupt the formation or function of composite cells [26, 27].

4.9 Potential for host-directed therapies

In addition to directly targeting the fungus, understanding composite cell formation may lead to host-directed therapies. These therapies could involve modulating the host's cellular processes to prevent integrating fungal elements, enhancing the host's ability to recognize and eliminate infected cells, or altering the host environment to make it less conducive to fungal survival [28].

The formation of composite cells in fungal infections represents a significant shift in our understanding of fungal pathogenesis. It challenges existing paradigms and demands a reevaluation of diagnostic and therapeutic approaches. As research continues to unravel the complexities of these interactions, it is poised to transform how we study, diagnose, and treat fungal diseases [29].

5. Evolutionary consi derations

The discovery of composite cells, particularly those involving *Aspergillus sydowii* and human keratinocytes, prompts a reexamination of the evolutionary strategies employed by pathogenic fungi. This section will explore the potential evolutionary considerations that may have led to the development of such a unique and complex interaction between fungi and their hosts.

5.1 Evolutionary pressures leading to intracellular survival

The evolution of pathogenic fungi involves a continuous arms race with their hosts, where both parties are under selective pressure to develop new survival strategies. The ability of certain fungi to survive and even thrive within host cells may have evolved in response to the host's immune defenses and antifungal treatments. This adaptation allows the fungus to persist in an environment where extracellular counterparts would be quickly eliminated [30].

5.2 The concept of parasitism and symbiosis in fungi

The formation of composite cells blurs the line between parasitism and symbiosis. While parasitism typically harms the host, the symbiotic relationship seen in composite cells suggests a level of cooperation or tolerance. This could indicate an evolutionary path where the fungus and host cell have reached a delicate balance, allowing the fungus to utilize the host's resources without immediately causing harm [31].

5.3 The role of genetic drift and selection in fungal pathogenesis

Genetic drift and natural selection play significant roles in the evolution of fungal pathogenesis. The emergence of composite cells may result from random genetic mutations that conferred a survival advantage within host tissues. Over time, these advantageous traits would be selected, leading to the prevalence of strains capable of forming composite cells within a population [32].

5.4 Co-evolution with the host immune system

The host immune system is a major driving force in the evolution of fungal pathogens. The ability of *Aspergillus sydowii* to form composite cells may be a coevolutionary response to the host's defenses. By integrating with human cells, the fungus may avoid detection by the immune system, representing an advanced strategy in the ongoing coevolutionary conflict [33].

5.5 The evolutionary trade-offs of intracellular lifestyle

The intracellular lifestyle of the fungus within composite cells may involve trade-offs. While offering protection from the host's immune system, it may also limit the fungus's ability to reproduce and spread. The evolution of mechanisms that allow the fungus to transition between intracellular and extracellular states could be a key factor in this strategy's success [34, 35].

5.6 Horizontal gene transfer and the acquisition of novel traits

Horizontal gene transfer (HGT) could play a role in evolving pathogenic traits in fungi. The ability to form composite cells may have been acquired through HGT from other intracellular pathogens, allowing *Aspergillus sydowii* to exploit a new ecological niche within the host [36, 37].

5.7 The impact of environmental factors on fungal evolution

Environmental factors, including changes in temperature, humidity, and nutrient availability, can influence the evolution of fungal pathogens. The adaptation to form composite cells may have been favored in environments where the host's immune defenses are robust, leading to the selection of fungal strains that can survive intracellularly [38, 39].

5.8 The evolution of virulence factors

The evolution of virulence factors in fungi is complex, involving the pathogen's ability to cause disease and evade host defenses. The formation of composite cells may represent a novel virulence factor that has evolved to enhance the pathogen's survival within the host [40].

5.9 Speciation and the role of composite cells in fungal diversity

The ability to form composite cells could influence the speciation of fungi. Different strains or species of *Aspergillus* may have varying abilities to form these cells, leading to distinct ecological roles and potentially driving speciation within the genus [41, 42].

5.10 Future directions in evolutionary research

Future research should aim to uncover the evolutionary history of the ability to form composite cells. This could involve comparative genomic studies to identify genes associated with this trait, phylogenetic analyses to trace the emergence of this capability, and experimental evolution studies to understand the selective pressures that favor its development [43].

The formation of composite cells by *Aspergillus sydowii* within human keratinocytes offers a unique lens through which to examine the evolutionary strategies of pathogenic fungi. Understanding the evolutionary considerations behind this phenomenon can provide valuable insights into fungal pathogenesis and inform the development of new therapeutic approaches. As our knowledge of fungal evolution grows, so too will our ability to predict and counteract the emergence of novel pathogenic strategies [44].

6. Pathogenesis and clinical manifestations of the Xiangya Lesion

The Xiangya Lesion, characterized by composite cells formed by *Aspergillus sydowii* and human keratinocytes, presents a unique challenge in understanding fungal infection pathogenesis. This section delves into the pathogenesis of the Xiangya Lesion and its clinical manifestations, providing a comprehensive overview of how these lesions develop and the signs and symptoms they present.

6.1 Pathogenesis of the Xiangya Lesion

The pathogenesis of the Xiangya Lesion is multifaceted, involving several steps that culminate in hyperkeratotic lesions.

6.1.1 Colonization and penetration

The process begins with *Aspergillus sydowii* colonizing the skin, potentially facilitated by microtraumas or preexisting skin conditions [45]. The fungus then penetrates the stratum corneum, encountering the keratinocytes.

6.1.2 Invasion and integration

Aspergillus sydowii exhibits invasive characteristics, allowing it to integrate with keratinocytes, forming anucleated composite cells [46, 47]. This integration is hypothesized to involve the release of fungal effector molecules that modulate host cell functions, leading to "zombie-like" cells that maintain some keratinocyte functions while expressing fungal characteristics.

6.1.3 Proliferation and overgrowth

The composite cells contribute to the Xiangya Lesion's pathogenesis through uncontrolled proliferation and overgrowth [3]. This abnormal cellular growth results in skin thickening, leading to the characteristic hyperkeratotic lesions. The overgrowth may be driven by fungal components within the composite cells, disrupting normal cell cycle regulation.

6.1.4 Immune evasion and persistence

A key pathogenic feature of the Xiangya Lesion is the composite cells' ability to evade the host's immune response [3]. The fungal elements are effectively shielded within the host cells, making them less susceptible to immune recognition and clearance. This immune evasion significantly contributes to the lesions' persistence and recurrence.

6.2 Clinical manifestations

6.2.1 Hyperkeratotic lesions

The primary clinical manifestation of the Xiangya Lesion is the presence of hyperkeratotic lesions on the plantar regions of the feet [3]. These lesions are often thick, hard, and may be accompanied by fissuring or cracking.

6.2.2 Patient discomfort

Patients may report discomfort, pain, and a feeling of heavy or stiff skin in the affected areas.

6.3 Diagnostic challenges

6.3.1 Atypical presentation

Diagnosing the Xiangya Lesion can be challenging due to its atypical presentation and the difficulty in detecting fungal elements within the composite cells.

6.3.2 Limitations of traditional methods

Traditional fungal culture methods may fail to isolate the pathogen if it is primarily intracellular.

6.3.3 Advanced techniques

Advanced diagnostic techniques, such as polymerase chain reaction (PCR) for fungal DNA or specific immunohistochemical staining, may be required for accurate diagnosis [3, 48].

6.4 Treatment considerations

6.4.1 Unique pathogenesis

Treatment of the Xiangya Lesion must consider the condition's unique pathogenesis.

6.4.2 Limited efficacy of standard treatments

Standard antifungal treatments may be less effective due to the pathogen's intracellular nature.

6.4.3 Combination therapies

Combination therapies targeting both the fungal and host cell components of the composite cells may be necessary.

6.4.4 Future directions

Treatments aimed at modulating the host's immune response or disrupting the formation of composite cells are areas of active investigation.

6.5 Clinical challenges

6.5.1 Recurrence and chronicity

The recurrence and chronicity of the Xiangya Lesion are significant clinical concerns. The fungus's ability to persist within host cells and the difficulty in completely eradicating the infection contributes to high relapse rates. Long-term management strategies and prophylactic measures are essential to reduce the risk of recurrence.

6.5.2 Impact on patient quality of life

The Xiangya Lesion can significantly impact a patient's quality of life [3]. The physical discomfort and cosmetic appearance of the lesions can lead to reduced mobility, social stigma, and psychological distress. Addressing these factors as part of a comprehensive treatment plan is crucial.

6.6 Future directions in research and treatment

6.6.1 Molecular mechanisms

Future research into the Xiangya Lesion should focus on elucidating the molecular mechanisms underlying the formation of composite cells and the pathogenesis of the lesions.

6.6.2 Targeted therapies and prevention

This knowledge can inform the development of targeted therapies and preventive strategies.

DOI: http://dx.doi.org/10.5772/intechopen.1005909

6.6.3 Epidemiology

Research into the epidemiology of the Xiangya Lesion can help identify risk factors and improve our understanding of its prevalence and distribution.

Conclusion: The Xiangya Lesion, with its complex pathogenesis and clinical manifestations, represents a significant challenge in dermatology and mycology. Understanding the intricate interplay between the host and the pathogen is key to developing effective diagnostic, treatment, and prevention strategies. As our knowledge of this condition grows, so too will our ability to manage and ultimately cure these challenging lesions.

7. Clinical and therapeutic implications

The Xiangya Lesion's clinical presentation often mimics other dermatological conditions, complicating diagnosis and necessitating a reevaluation of current diagnostic and treatment protocols for fungal infections. This section explores the challenges faced in clinical practice and proposes potential therapeutic strategies that may be effective against the Xiangya Lesion's unique pathogenesis.

7.1 Clinical presentation and diagnosis

7.1.1 Mimicking other conditions

Patients with the Xiangya Lesion typically exhibit plantar hyperkeratosis, which can be mistaken for common calluses or other noninfectious skin conditions.

7.1.2 High index of suspicion

Accurate diagnosis requires a high index of suspicion.

7.1.3 Advanced diagnostic techniques

Diagnosis may involve advanced diagnostic techniques such as skin biopsies, histological examination, and molecular identification of the fungal pathogen.

7.2 Diagnostic challenges and solutions

7.2.1 Intracellular nature of the pathogen

The intracellular nature of *Aspergillus sydowii* within the Xiangya Lesion presents a significant diagnostic challenge. Traditional fungal cultures may fail to detect the pathogen if it is not extracellularly released.

7.2.2 Molecular diagnostics

The use of molecular diagnostic methods, such as PCR, can detect the presence of fungal DNA within the composite cells, offering a more sensitive and specific diagnostic approach.

7.3 Antifungal resistance and treatment failures

7.3.1 Resistance to conventional treatments

The resistance of the Xiangya Lesion to conventional antifungal treatments is a major clinical concern. The intracellular location of the fungus may shield it from antifungal drugs that typically target extracellular fungal elements.

7.3.2 Understanding resistance mechanisms

Understanding the mechanisms of resistance is crucial for developing new therapeutic strategies.

7.4 Potential therapeutic approaches

7.4.1 Novel drug development

Given the unique pathogenesis of the Xiangya Lesion, novel therapeutic approaches are necessary. This may involve developing drugs that can penetrate host cells and target intracellular fungi.

7.4.2 Immunomodulation

Therapies that modulate the host's immune response to better recognize and eliminate the composite cells could be beneficial.

7.5 Specific therapeutic strategies

7.5.1 Immunomodulatory therapies

Immunomodulatory therapies that enhance the host's immune response against the fungal pathogen maybe a promising avenue for treatment. This could involve using cytokines, immune-stimulating complexes, or other agents that boost the host's ability to clear the infection.

7.5.2 Combination therapies

Combination therapies targeting both the fungal and host components of the composite cells may be more effective than single-agent treatment]. This could involve combining antifungal drugs with different mechanisms of action and agents that disrupt the host-fungus interaction.

7.5.3 Host-directed therapies

Host-directed therapies aim to alter the host environment to make it less conducive to fungal survival and proliferation [39]. This could involve treatments that inhibit the formation of composite cells or promote the host's natural cell turnover to remove infected cells.

7.5.4 Surgical interventions

In some cases, surgical interventions may be necessary to manage Xiangya Lesion, particularly when conservative treatments have failed [40]. Surgical options could include debridement of the affected tissue or more extensive procedures to remove larger areas of infected skin.

7.6 Patient management and public health

7.6.1 Patient education and compliance

Educating patients about the nature of the Xiangya Lesion, its treatment, and the importance of compliance with therapy is critical. Given the chronic and relapsing nature of the condition, patients must understand the long-term management and the need for ongoing monitoring and care.

7.6.2 Preventive measures

Preventive measures are essential to reduce the risk of developing the Xiangya Lesion. This could involve maintaining good foot hygiene, wearing appropriate footwear, and avoiding environments that may predispose to fungal infections.

7.6.3 Future research directions

Future research should focus on understanding the molecular and cellular mechanisms underlying the formation and persistence of the Xiangya Lesion. This knowledge can inform the development of targeted therapies and preventive strategies. Additionally, research into the epidemiology and risk factors for the Xiangya Lesion can help identify those most at risk and guide public health initiatives.

Conclusion: The clinical and therapeutic implications of the Xiangya Lesion are complex and require a multifaceted approach to management. As our understanding of this condition grows, so too will our ability to develop effective treatments and improve patient outcomes. It is through continued research and innovation that we will ultimately overcome the challenges posed by this intriguing and clinically significant fungal pathogenesis.

8. Future research directions

The discovery of the Xiangya Lesion and the unique pathogenesis of *Aspergillus sydowii* within human keratinocytes opens up a new frontier in medical mycology and dermatology. Future research should aim to elucidate the underlying mechanisms, improve diagnostics, and develop novel therapeutic strategies.

8.1 Molecular mechanisms of infection

A detailed understanding of how *Aspergillus sydowii* infects and integrates with human keratinocytes is crucial. Research should focus on:

1. Identifying the fungal and host factors involved in forming composite cells.

2. Investigating the role of fungal effector proteins and host cell receptors in this process [49].

8.2 Immunological response to infection

The host's immunological response to the Xiangya Lesion is a key area for future research. Studies should investigate:

1. How the host's immune system recognizes and responds to the infection.

2. How the fungus evades or manipulates these defenses.

3. The potential for developing immunotherapies that enhance the host's ability to clear the infection [50].

8.3 Genetic and epigenetic factors

Research into the genetic and epigenetic factors influencing susceptibility to and progression of the Xiangya Lesion is essential. This may include studying:

1. Genetic variations among individuals that affect their response to the infection.

2. Epigenetic changes within host cells due to fungal integration.

8.4 Evolutionary biology of aspergillus sydowii

The evolutionary biology of *Aspergillus sydowii*, particularly its ability to form composite cells, is a fascinating area for exploration.

1. Comparative genomics and phylogenetic analyses can provide insights into the evolutionary pressures that led to this adaptation and its prevalence among other fungal species [51].

8.5 Development of new diagnostic tools

Developing new diagnostic tools for accurate and efficient Xiangya Lesion detection is critical. This may involve:

1. Creating new molecular assays, imaging techniques, or biomarkers specific to the infection [52].

8.6 Novel antifungal agents

Given the resistance of the Xiangya Lesion to conventional antifungal treatments, developing new antifungal agents is imperative. These should:

1. Target the unique aspects of the infection, such as the fungal components within composite cells.

2. Disrupt the mechanisms allowing the fungus to proliferate within the host [53].

8.7 Host-directed therapies

Research into host-directed therapies that alter the host environment to hinder fungal survival is another promising avenue. This may include treatments that:

1. Inhibit the formation of composite cells.

2. Enhance the host's natural cell turnover to eliminate infected cells.

8.8 Immunomodulatory approaches

Immunomodulatory approaches that enhance the host's immune response to the infection are a significant area for future research. This may involve using:

1. Cytokines, toll-like receptor agonists, or other immune-stimulating agents that boost the host's ability to recognize and clear infected cells [54].

8.9 Impact of environmental factors

The impact of environmental factors on the development and progression of the Xiangya Lesion should be investigated. This can include studying the role of:

1. Temperature, humidity, and other environmental conditions on the growth and spread of the infection [3, 14].

8.10 Clinical trials and treatment protocols

Clinical trials to evaluate the efficacy and safety of new treatments for the Xiangya Lesion are essential. This should involve:

1. Developing standardized treatment protocols and outcome measures to assess the success of these therapies.

8.11 Epidemiological studies

Epidemiological studies are needed to determine:

1. The prevalence, risk factors, and geographic distribution of the Xiangya Lesion.

2. This information can inform public health strategies and guide resource allocation for prevention and treatment [54].

8.12 Education and awareness

Increasing awareness about the Xiangya Lesion among healthcare professionals and the general public is critical. Educational initiatives should focus on:

1. The signs, symptoms, and transmission of the infection.

2. The importance of early diagnosis and treatment.

3. Early diagnosis and treatment of Aspergillus infection may prevent Xiangya Lesion formation.

8.13 Interdisciplinary collaboration

Future research should encourage interdisciplinary collaboration between:

1. Dermatologists, mycologists, immunologists, geneticists, and other relevant fields.

2. This collaborative approach can lead to a more comprehensive understanding of Xiangya Lesion and the development of more effective treatment strategies.

Conclusion: The Xiangya Lesion represents a significant challenge in medical mycology and dermatology. Future research should build on the current understanding of this condition, focusing on molecular mechanisms, immunological responses, genetic factors, and developing novel diagnostic and therapeutic tools. Through continued research and collaboration, significant strides can be made in managing and ultimately curing this complex fungal infection.

9. Conclusion

The exploration of the Xiangya Lesion and its implications for fungal pathogenesis has revealed a complex and intriguing landscape of host-fungus interactions. *Aspergillus sydowii*'s ability to form composite cells with human keratinocytes has profound implications for our understanding of fungal infections, their diagnosis, and treatment.

9.1 Synergistic pathogenesis

The Xiangya Lesion's pathogenesis is a synergistic process where the fungus and host cell coalesce into the "zombie cell." This phenomenon challenges traditional pathogenesis models and suggests a more nuanced view of host-pathogen interactions, blurring the line between self and nonself.

9.2 Diagnostic innovations

The diagnostic challenges presented by the Xiangya Lesion necessitate developing innovative diagnostic tools. Molecular techniques like PCR and DNA sequencing have proven invaluable in identifying the fungal presence within composite cells. Future research may uncover additional biomarkers or imaging techniques to detect these unique cells specifically.

9.3 Therapeutic advances

The Xiangya Lesion's resistance to conventional antifungal therapies has spurred the search for new treatment modalities. This includes developing drugs that target intracellular pathogens, immunomodulatory therapies to enhance the host's immune response and host-directed therapies that disrupt the formation of composite cells.

9.4 Evolutionary insights

The evolutionary considerations of the Xiangya Lesion provide a framework for understanding how *Aspergillus sydowii* has adapted to survive within the host. Further research into this fungus's evolutionary biology may reveal additional strategies employed to evade host defenses and establish a persistent infection.

9.5 Clinical management

Managing the Xiangya Lesion clinically requires a multidisciplinary approach involving dermatologists, mycologists, immunologists, and other specialists. Developing standardized treatment protocols and patient education initiatives will be critical in improving patient outcomes.

9.6 Public health implications

The public health implications of the Xiangya Lesion extend beyond individual patient care. Understanding the epidemiology of this condition – its prevalence, risk factors, and geographic distribution – is essential for informing public health strategies for prevention and control.

9.7 Research priorities

Future research priorities should include:

1. A deeper investigation into the molecular dialog between *Aspergillus sydowii* and human keratinocytes.

2. * Developing new diagnostic and therapeutic tools.

3. * Implementing clinical trials to evaluate the efficacy of these innovations.

9.8 Interdisciplinary collaboration

The complexity of the Xiangya Lesion demands an interdisciplinary approach to research and clinical practice. Collaboration between biologists, clinicians, and public health professionals will be key to advancing our understanding of this condition and improving patient care.

9.9 Knowledge dissemination

Disseminating knowledge about the Xiangya Lesion to the scientific community and the general public is critical. This includes publishing research findings in peer-reviewed journals, presenting at scientific conferences, and engaging in public education campaigns.

9.10 Ethical considerations

Ethical considerations in research and patient care are paramount, particularly when considering novel diagnostic and therapeutic techniques.

1. Ensuring research is conducted ethically and patients are fully informed about their treatment options is essential.

9.11 Long-term vision

The long-term vision for Xiangya Lesion research is to develop a comprehensive understanding of this condition, from its molecular underpinnings to its clinical manifestations. This knowledge will inform the development of effective treatments and, ultimately, the prevention of the disease.

In conclusion, the Xiangya Lesion represents a significant advancement in our understanding of fungal pathogenesis. The research presented here has broad implications for medical mycology and the potential to transform how we diagnose and treat fungal infections. As we continue to unravel the complexities of this condition, we move closer to a future where the challenges posed by the Xiangya Lesion are effectively managed and, hopefully, eradicated.

Acknowledgements

The author acknowledges the use of Claude 3 for language polishing of the manuscript.

Conflict of interest

The authors declare no conflict of interest.

Author details

Xiujuan Yan[1] and Charles Xiaoxiang Zhu[2*]

1 Institute of Clinical Pharmacology, Central South University, Changsha, China

2 Xiangya Medical School, Changsha, China

*Address all correspondence to: charles.zhu@live.com

References

[1] Heilmann-Clausen J, Barron E, Boddy L, Dahlberg A, Griffith G, Nordén J, et al. A fungal perspective on conservation biology. Conservation Biology. 2015;**29**:61-68. DOI: 10.1111/cobi.12388

[2] Yakop F, Taha H, Shivanand P. Isolation of fungi from various habitats and their possible bioremediation. Current Science. 2019;**116**(5):733-740. DOI: 10.18520/cs/v116/i5/733-740

[3] Zhu C, Li X, Tan X, Wu G. Zombie cells, composite cells of fungal–human keratinocytes of plantar hyperkeratosis-like lesions. Mycopathologia. 2019;**184**:597-605. DOI: 10.1007/s11046-019-00369-0

[4] Spink M, Menz H, Lord S. Distribution and correlates of plantar hyperkeratotic lesions in older people. Journal of Foot and Ankle Research. 2009;**2**:8-8. DOI: 10.1186/1757-1146-2-8

[5] Freeman DB. Corns and calluses resulting from mechanical hyperkeratosis. American Family Physician. 2002;**65**(11):2277-2280

[6] Pereiro et al. Plantar hyperkeratosis due to Fusarium verticillioides in a patient with malignancy. Clinical and Experimental Dermatology. 1999;**24**:175-178. DOI: 10.1046/j.1365-2230.1999.00447.x

[7] Rothman S et al. Systemic disturbances in recalcitrant trichophyton rubrum (purpureum) infections; studies and short report on therapeutic experiments. A.M.A. Archives of Dermatology and Syphilology. 1953;**67**(3):239-246. DOI: 10.1001/ARCHDERM.1953.01540030002001

[8] Scorzoni L, Silva A, Marcos C, Assato P, Melo W, Oliveira H, et al. Antifungal therapy: New advances in the understanding and treatment of mycosis. Frontiers in Microbiology. 2017;**8**:36. DOI: 10.3389/fmicb.2017.00036

[9] Hopsu-Havu V, Sonck C, Tunnela E. Production of elastase by pathogenic and non-pathogenic fungi. Mycoses. 1972;**15**:105-110. DOI: 10.1111/j.1439-0507.1972.tb01357.x

[10] Cooney N, Klein B. Fungal adaptation to the mammalian host: It is a new world, after all. Current Opinion in Microbiology. 2008;**11**(6):511-516. DOI: 10.1016/j.mib.2008.09.018

[11] Cornejo E, Schlaermann P, Mukherjee S. How to rewire the host cell: A home improvement guide for intracellular bacteria. The Journal of Cell Biology. 2017;**216**:3931-3948. DOI: 10.1083/jcb.201701095

[12] Arunachalam D, Namperumalsamy V, Prajna L, Kuppamuthu D. Human corneal epithelial cells internalize aspergillus flavus spores by actin-mediated endocytosis. Infection and Immunity. 2021;**89**(6):e00794-e00820. DOI: 10.1128/IAI.00794-20

[13] Pandey A, Ding S, Qin Q, Gupta R, Gomez G, Lin F, et al. Global reprogramming of host kinase Signaling in response to fungal infection. Cell Host & Microbe. 2017;**21**(5):637-649.e6. DOI: 10.1016/j.chom.2017.04.008

[14] Zhu CX. Season, weather, arthritis, dermatitis and cardiovascular abnormalities—a case of systemic diseases caused by fungal foot infection and its secreted proteins. 2018. DOI: 10.13140/rg.2.2.11508.60807. Available

from: https://www.researchgate.net/publication/329906487. [Accessed: January 18, 2019]

[15] Souza J, Gurgel I, Malacco N, Martins F, Queiroz-Junior C, Teixeira M, et al. Pre-exposure with extracellular vesicles from aspergillus fumigatus attenuates inflammatory response and enhances fungal clearance in a murine model pulmonary Aspergillosis. Frontiers in Cellular and Infection Microbiology. 2022;**12**:898619. DOI: 10.3389/fcimb.2022.898619

[16] Lima S, Colombo A, Júnior J. Fungal Cell Wall: Emerging antifungals and drug resistance. Frontiers in Microbiology. 2019;**10**:2573. DOI: 10.3389/fmicb.2019.02573

[17] Hasim S, Coleman J. Targeting the fungal cell wall: Current therapies and implications for development of alternative antifungal agents. Future Medicinal Chemistry. 2019;**11**(8):869-883. DOI: 10.4155/fmc-2018-0465

[18] Hernández-Chávez M, Pérez-García L, Niño-Vega G, Mora-Montes H. Fungal strategies to evade the host immune recognition. Journal of Fungi. 2017;**3**:51. DOI: 10.3390/jof3040051

[19] Crawford A, Wilson D. Essential metals at the host–pathogen interface: Nutritional immunity and micronutrient assimilation by human fungal pathogens. FEMS Yeast Research. 2015;**15**(7):fov071. DOI: 10.1093/femsyr/fov071

[20] Erwig L, Gow N. Interactions of fungal pathogens with phagocytes. Nature Reviews Microbiology. 2016;**14**:163-176. DOI: 10.1038/nrmicro.2015.21

[21] Romani L. The T cell response against fungal infections. Current Opinion in Immunology. 1997;**9**(4):484-490. DOI: 10.1016/S0952-7915(97)80099-4

[22] García-Carnero L, Martínez-Álvarez J, Salazar-García L, Lozoya-Pérez N, González-Hernández S, Tamez-Castrellón A. Recognition of fungal components by the host immune system. Current Protein & Peptide Science. 2019;**21**(3):245-264. DOI: 10.2174/138920372 1666191231105546

[23] Hopke A, Brown A, Hall R, Wheeler R. Dynamic fungal Cell Wall architecture in stress adaptation and immune evasion. Trends in Microbiology. 2018;**26**(4):284-295. DOI: 10.1016/j.tim.2018.01.007

[24] Cohen M, Istùriz R, Malech H, Root R, Wilfert C, Gutman L, et al. Fungal infection in chronic granulomatous disease. The importance of the phagocyte in defense against fungi. The American Journal of Medicine. 1981;**71**(1):59-66. DOI: 10.1016/0002-9343(81)90259-X

[25] Wuyts J, Dijck P, Holtappels M. Fungal persister cells: The basis for recalcitrant infections? PLoS Pathogens. 2018;**14**(10):e1007301. DOI: 10.1371/journal.ppat.1007301

[26] Min K, Neiman A, Konopka J. Fungal pathogens: Shape-shifting invaders. Trends in Microbiology. 2020(11):922-933. DOI: 10.1016/j.tim.2020.05.001

[27] Casadevall A. Evolution of intracellular pathogens. Annual Review of Microbiology. 2008;**62**:19-33. DOI: 10.1146/annurev.micro.61.080706.093305

[28] Klepzig K, Adams A, Handelsman J, Raffa K. Symbioses: A key driver of insect physiological processes, ecological interactions. Evolutionary

Diversification, and Impacts on Humans*. 2009;**38**:67-77. DOI: 10.1603/022.038.0109

[29] Stukenbrock E, Croll D. The evolving fungal genome. Fungal Biology Reviews. 2014;**28**:1-12. DOI: 10.1016/J.FBR.2014.02.001

[30] Lovero K, Treseder K. Trade-offs between growth rate and other fungal traits. Frontiers in Forests and Global Change. 2021;**4**:756650. DOI: 10.3389/ffgc.2021.756650

[31] Woodhams D, Alford R, Briggs C, Johnson M, Rollins-Smith L. Life-history trade-offs influence disease in changing climates: Strategies of an amphibian pathogen. Ecology. 2008;**89**(6):1627-1639. DOI: 10.1890/06-1842.1

[32] Ademe M. Immunomodulation for the treatment of fungal infections: Opportunities and challenges. Frontiers in Cellular and Infection Microbiology. 2020;**10**:469. DOI: 10.3389/fcimb.2020.00469

[33] Armstrong-James D, Brown G, Netea M, Zelante T, Gresnigt M, Veerdonk F, et al. Immunotherapeutic approaches to treatment of fungal diseases. The Lancet. Infectious diseases. 2017;**17**(12):e393-e402. DOI: 10.1016/S1473-3099(17)30442-5

[34] Williams T, Harvey S, Armstrong-James D. Immunotherapeutic approaches for fungal infections. Current Opinion in Microbiology. 2020;**58**:130-137. DOI: 10.1016/j.mib.2020.09.007

[35] Gustafson E, Bakotic W, Bennett L, Page L, McCarthy L. DNA-based detection for onychomycosis correlates better to histopathology than does fungal culture. Dermatology Online Journal. 2019;**25**:7. DOI: 10.5070/D3257044800

[36] Nie X, Li B, Wang S. Epigenetic and posttranslational modifications in regulating the biology of aspergillus species. Advances in Applied Microbiology. 2018;**105**:191-226. DOI: 10.1016/bs.aambs.2018.05.004

[37] Procop G. Molecular diagnostics for the detection and characterization of microbial pathogens. Clinical infectious diseases: an official publication of the Infectious Diseases Society of America. 2007;**45**(Suppl. 2):S99-S111. DOI: 10.1086/519259

[38] Filler S, Sheppard D. Fungal invasion of normally non-phagocytic host cells. PLoS Pathogens. 2006;**2**(2):e129. DOI: 10.1371/journal.ppat.0020129

[39] Sonnex C. Toll-like receptors and genital tract infection. International Journal of STD & AIDS. 2010;**21**:153-157. DOI: 10.1258/ijsa.2009.009525

[40] Barbosa E, Gonçalves A, Guerra M, Cruz C. A systematic review on resource allocation in public health. European Journal of Public Health. 2020;**30**:v1018-v1019. DOI: 10.1093/eurpub/ckaa166.1309

[41] Giraud T, Refrégier G, Mickael Le G, et al. Speciation in fungi. Fungal Genetics and Biology: FG & B. 2008;**45**(6):791-802. DOI: 10.1016/j.fgb.2008.02.001

[42] Meredith DMJ, Irene F, Gadelha C, et al. Discovery of novel intermediate forms redefines the fungal tree of life. Nature. 2011;**474**:200-203. DOI: 10.1038/nature09984

[43] Alshehri B, Palanisamy M. Evaluation of molecular identification of Aspergillus species causing fungal keratitis. Saudi Journal of Biological Sciences. 2019;**27**:751-756. DOI: 10.1016/j.sjbs.2019.12.030

[44] Parismita B, Barua P, Pranjal Jyoti D, et al. Onychomycosis associated with superficial skin infection due to Aspergillus sydowii in an immunocompromised patient. Mycopathologia. 2019;**184**:683-689. DOI: 10.1007/s11046-019-00383-2

[45] Themistoklis KK, Fuchs B, Jeffrey JC, et al. Polymerase chain reaction-based assays for the diagnosis of invasive fungal infections. Clinical Infectious Diseases: An Official Publication of the Infectious Diseases Society of America. 2012;**54**(9):1322-1331. DOI: 10.1093/cid/cis132

[46] McCarthy M, Walsh T. PCR methodology and applications for the detection of human fungal pathogens. Expert Review of Molecular Diagnostics. 2016;**16**:1025-1036. DOI: 10.1080/14737159.2016.1219253

[47] Alexandra NM, Jeffery U, Zachary GS, et al. Diagnostic accuracy of a direct panfungal polymerase chain reaction assay performed on stained cytology slides. Veterinary Pathology. 2021;**58**:542-548. DOI: 10.1177/0300985821991562

[48] Criven J, Tenforde M, Levitz S, et al. Modulating host immune responses to fight invasive fungal infections. Current Opinion in Microbiology. 2017;**40**:95-103. DOI: 10.1016/j.mib.2017.10.018

[49] Fisher R, Bridget G, Helaine S. Persistent bacterial infections and persister cells. Nature Reviews Microbiology. 2017;**15**:453-464. DOI: 10.1038/nrmicro.2017.42

[50] Sipsas N, Kontoyiannis D. Clinical issues regarding relapsing aspergillosis and the efficacy of secondary antifungal prophylaxis in patients with hematological malignancies. Clinical Infectious Diseases: An Official Publication of the Infectious Diseases Society of America. 2006;**42**(11): 1584-1591. DOI: 10.1086/503844

[51] Georgopapadakou N, Jan ST. The fungal cell wall as a drug target. Trends in Microbiology. 1995;**3**(3):98-104. DOI: 10.1016/S0966-842X(00)88890-3

[52] Kung V, Chernock R, Burnham C. Diagnostic accuracy of fungal identification in histopathology and cytopathology specimens. European Journal of Clinical Microbiology & Infectious Diseases. 2017;**37**:157-165. DOI: 10.1007/s10096-017-3116-3

[53] Kanafani Z, Perfect J. Resistance to antifungal agents: Mechanisms and clinical impact. Clinical Infectious Diseases. 2008;**46**:120-128. DOI: 10.1086/524071

[54] Bossche HV, Marichal P, Odds FC. Molecular mechanisms of drug resistance in fungi. Trends in Microbiology. 1994;**2**(10):393-400. DOI: 10.1016/0966-842X(94)90618-1

Section 4

Mycorrhizal Fungi

Chapter 8

Arbuscular Mycorrhizal Fungi and Magnetically Treated Water in the Biocontrol of Nematodes: Experiences in Protected Cultivation Technology

Daniel Rafael Vuelta Lorenzo, Siannah María Más Diego, Gerardo Montero Limonta and Miriela Rizo Mustelier

Abstract

Cuban agriculture works on a general agroecological pest management scheme, where biological control is of great importance. Traditionally, arbuscular mycorrhizal fungi (AMF) have been considered as biofertilizers, undervaluing their potential for plant protection. The objective of this research was to evaluate the effect of AMF as a biological control agent of *Meloidogyne incognita* in combination with irrigation with magnetically treated water (MTW) in protected cultivation. It was carried out in the Campo Antena protected cultivation unit in Santiago de Cuba, Cuba, in the tomato, pepper, cucumber and chard crops. It was determined that AMF inoculation combined with MTW is viable to manage *M. incognita* populations, in vegetables under protected cultivation conditions, achieving an increase in yields and a decrease in nematode populations. This work supports the results obtained from the selection of promising strains given the type of existing soil. In addition, it provides practical elements that make up a modified methodology for the use of AMF + MTW in the management of nematodes in intensive vegetable production systems under protected cultivation conditions.

Keywords: *Meloidogyne incognita*, microorganism, biologic control, magnetic induction, greenhouse

1. Introduction

Modern, industrial, conventional or green revolution agriculture is in crisis and affects the economy of all countries in the world. The effects are socioeconomic and ecological in nature, which means that producers cannot cope with the high price of modern products and technologies. On the other hand, its effect is manifested in the progressive decrease in agricultural yields, in addition to the loss of biodiversity [1, 2].

The indiscriminate use of pesticides affects the population of beneficial insects and has caused pest resistance. An attempt has been made to alleviate this situation with the mixture of more toxic products that, although they can temporarily solve the problem, result in new resistance, resurgence, outbreak of secondary pests and a decrease in natural enemies [3].

Plant-parasitic nematodes are associated with effects on the development and production of agricultural crops, being recognized as one of the limiting factors in yields [4]. Among root-knot nematodes such as *Meloidogyne incognita* (Kofoid and White), Chitwood is the species most commonly found on vegetables. Plant-parasitic nematodes are associated with effects on the development and production of agricultural crops, being recognized as one of the limiting factors in yields [4, 5], causing damage to numerous crops of agricultural interest.

The most important species in Cuba is *M. incognita*, and for its management various practices are used that include the use of biological control agents [6], and it constitutes one of the most important phytosanitary problems of horticultural crops [7]. The root-knot nematode, *Meloidogyne incognita*, is an emergent nematode in protected conditions. This nematode can cause chlorosis, stunted growth, and reduced host plant yields. Root-knot nematodes severely affect the root system of the plant by inducing the formation of specialized nutritional cells, that is, giant cells in the vascular tissues. Recently, this nematode has been considered as a global threat in protected cultivation technology [8].

Farmers apply pesticides due to the need to protect their crops, without taking into account the toxicity of the product, which leads to contamination of crops by chemical residues, which has repercussions on the soil, air and water [9]. Currently, alternatives to chemical control have been sought with the use of microorganisms and cultural practices that allow integrated management of nematodes [10].

Furthermore, it is important to point out the need to consider the health of plants and their microbiome within the "one health" concept, closely linked to the health of the environment, soil, animals and people. In the context of agroecological production based on the sustainable management of natural resources, integrated pest management has been promoted to reduce the use of pesticides and mitigate negative effects on human and environmental health. For this, biological control has contributed to achieving this goal [11].

Biological control applies to the use of living organisms, as AMF, to suppress the population density or impact of a specific pest organism. In this case, biological control of nematodes is manifested by the regulation of nematode populations or their damage through the action of antagonistic organisms, and this occurs naturally or through manipulation of the environment or the introduction of antagonists [12].

Arbuscular mycorrhizal fungi (AMF) constitute a functional group that is important in the soil biota, as it favors the improvement of the structure, the multifunctionality of the ecosystem and the productive development of crops [13]. The importance of the study of AMF lies in the fact that there is evidence of its association with more than 80% of plants, as well as its role in protecting the root system from phytopathogenic agents, promoting mineral nutrition and facilitating water absorption, which contributes to the improvement of plant growth and survival [14].

Effective management of mycorrhizal associations may be a means to increase the productivity of agricultural crops, as AMF are vital components of the rhizosphere of these crops. Plants maintain a close relationship through a network of interconnected hyphae that increase the area of soil explored by roots, improve their structure and facilitate the absorption of nutrients and water, among other essential functions. The effects of these microorganisms not only have consequences on development and nutrition but can also increase the natural resistance of plants in situations of biotic (pathogenic) or abiotic (water or saline stress) imbalances [15].

Although it can be applied in the field, with various restrictions, the main application of these fungi is in those systems that require a nursery phase, before they are released into the field. The management or establishment of the biotechnology represented by arbuscular mycorrhizal fungi (AMF) must be carried out in the first phases of the growth and/or establishment of the plants, so that they receive the greatest benefit prior to their commercial exploitation in orchards [16]. There are several studies on the effects of AMF on plants attacked by nematodes [17], in most of which a decrease in the severity of the infestation is observed. The mechanisms are related to the contribution of resistance to the plant and in general depend on changes in the host's physiology. Changes in root exudates would modify the attraction of nematodes to the roots [18].

Mycorrhiza-forming fungi provide innumerable benefits for the plant and services for the functioning of the ecosystem, contribute to plant nutrition, health and water balance and generate a network of mycelium in the soil, through which the roots communicate with each other and share information, water and nutrients. This network is a valuable way to conserve soil carbon and nutrients (these are considered ecosystem services). Furthermore, mycorrhizae are involved in the production of a binding substance for soil particles that favors the formation of aggregates and reduces the risk of erosion [19].

The use of the magnetic field (CM) influences microbial growth, either inhibiting it or stimulating it, and this depends on the intensity and time of exposure. The effect of CM on microbial growth is not only one, and it can be classified as unobservable, inhibitory and stimulatory [20].

In Cuba, there is the National Center of Applied Magnetism (CNEA) which is a multidisciplinary institution with the purpose of researching and applying magnetic and electromagnetic fields in industry, medicine, agriculture and the environment, and in its work, it has carried out numerous investigations in agriculture demonstrating the positive effects of magnetically treated water (MTW) on crops [21–23]. There are few studies that propose the use of MTW to combat pests, specifically nematodes, as plants subjected to magnetically treated water tend to behave tolerant to these pathogens [24–27], but information on its direct effect on nematode control is limited.

The technology of protected cultivation houses is a form of intensive agriculture that can contribute to local food security, its advantages are protection against extreme weather conditions, obtaining permanent crops through continuous sowing, better quality of the harvest, reduction of soil erosion, planting of selected materials, significant increase in yield, decrease in pest attack, due to physical barriers such as meshes, more efficient use of the growing area and opportunity to access new markets, due to the improvement in the safety of the crops products [28].

However, the high incidence of nematodes causes considerable damage to the production of protected crops. This situation limits producers from obtaining high yields from their crops and also implies a high cost for the use of chemical nematocides. Therefore, the objective was to evaluate the management of nematodes with the combined application of AMF and MTW, which allows reducing the impact to acceptable levels in protected cultivation conditions.

2. Use of arbuscular mycorrhizal fungi and magnetically treated water for the management of nematodes in protected culture conditions

The research was carried out in the municipality of Santiago de Cuba in the Protected Crop Unit in Campo Antena, of the Socialist State Company América Libre, and was carried out in the period from February 2018 to March 2021. The entity where the research was developed is located on the Santiago de Cuba; reference coordinate (X: 60757330 Y: 156332149). It has an area of 1.52 ha, with 23 cultivation houses that are used for the production of vegetables, such as pepper, tomato, chard and cucumber during the experiment period.

For the application of the treatments, a high-frequency localized irrigation system was implemented, which allowed the immediate application of water after magnetization. The experiments used external permanent magnet or static magnetic field devices, designed at the National Center for Applied Electromagnetism (CNEA).

A part of the water circulation pipe was placed at the two poles of the magnetizer, and the direction of water flow is perpendicular to the direction of the magnetic induction line. The magnetic inductions were set at 0.05–0.07 Tesla (T) and 0.1–0.12 T. The treatment was carried out at the time of watering the plants, throughout the crop cycle until development of the fruits. Irrigation was carried out once a day through a drip system, for 30 minutes. The conditions established for irrigation considered the water speed (1.4–1.6 m s^{-1}) and the pump flow (2.54–2.91 m^3 h^{-1}). The treated water began to be used immediately after transplanting and until the end of the experiment.

The experimental design was completely randomized, with four replications and 12 treatments.

Three strains of AMF were used in the research:

Rhizophagus irregularis (Błaszk., Wubet, Renker & Buscot), C. Walker & A. Schüßler.

Funneliformis mosseae (T.H. Nicolson & Gerd.), C. Walker & A. Schüßler.

Glomus cubense (Y. Rodr. Dalpé).

2.1 Forms of seed inoculation

For the treatment of the seeds, a homogeneous paste was prepared with water, in a proportion of 1 kg of each inoculum for every 10 kg of seed, and the seed was covered with it until it was completely covered according to the methodology [29]. The inoculated mixture was allowed to rest in the shade for 10 minutes, and then the seedbed was established.

The seeds were sown by treatments in polyfoam trays (expanded polyethylene), each with 150 truncated pyramidal alveoli, previously washed with soap and water and subsequent disinfection by immersion in chlorinated solution (concentration) or agricultural iodine (5 mL/L of water) [30]. The substrate was composed of worm castings (80%) and peat (20%).

Sowing was carried out manually, by depositing two to three seeds per socket at a depth of 2–3 mm. Subsequently, the trays were placed in the dark for three days. Then, they were moved to a protected area with a flexible polyethylene cover, anti-bemisia lateral meshes, and separated from the ground between 60 and 100 cm. Daily localized irrigation or with a watering can was maintained. **Table 1** shows the description of the treatments used in this research.

	Treatments
1	Control without inoculation of AMF
2	Culture without inoculation of AMF + MTW (0.05–0.07 T)
3	Culture without inoculation of AMF + MTW (0.1–0.12 T)
4	*Rhizophagus irregularis*
5	*Funneliformis mosseae*
6	*Glomus cubense*
7	*Rhizophagus irregularis* + MTW (0.05–0.07 T)
8	*Rhizophagus irregularis* + MTW (0.1–0.12 T)
9	*Funneliformis mosseae* + MTW (0.05–0.07 T)
10	*Funneliformis mosseae* + MTW (0.1–0.12 T)
11	*Glomus cubense* + MTW (0.05–0.07 T)
12	*Glomus cubense* + MTW (0.1–0.12 T)

Table 1.
Description of the treatments.

2.2 Tomato cultivation *(Solanum lycopersicum* L.)

The crop used was tomato (hybrid variety HA 3057) of determined growth. It was evaluated from transplant to final production. Four houses of 0.080 ha were used for a total experimental area of 0.22 ha, with a duration of 120 days. The planting frame was 1.04 m × 0.30 m.

2.3 The cultivation of pepper *(Capsicum annuum* L.)

The crop used was the Locumone hybrid variety pepper. It was evaluated from transplantation to final production. Four houses of 0.08 ha were used as the experimental area for a total experimental area of 0.32 ha. The duration of the crop cycle was 120 days.

2.4 Cultivation of cucumber *(Cucumis sativus* L.)

I grow indeterminate growing cucumber. Hybrid Variety YA 2005. The stage from transplanting root balls to final production was evaluated. The duration of the crop cycle was 120 days. The planting frame was 1.5 m × 0.30 m.

2.5 The cultivation of chard (*Beta vulgaris* var. *cicla* L.)

For this experiment, chard (improved variety PK – 7) was used as a crop. The period evaluated was from sowing to final production. Four cultivation houses of 0.054 ha were used for a total experimental area of 0.22 ha. The duration of the crop cycle was 45 days. The planting distance was 1.04 m × 0.25 m × 0.25 m from ridge to double furrow and 0.25 m from nose (two or three seeds per row). Optimum population density was 20–30 plants/m^2 at the bottom of the furrow.

For the agronomic management of the crops, we proceeded as stipulated by the Manual for the Protected Production of Vegetables [31].

2.6 Statistical analysis

For the comparison of treatments, simple classification analysis of variance was performed, and the means were compared by Tukey's multiple range test at a 5% probability. For non-parametric evaluations, the Kruskal-Wallis test was used. For each analysis, the assumptions of normality and homogeneity of variance were checked (Bartlett's test and Kolmogorov-Smirnov test, respectively) in each variable evaluated through the statistical program R commander version 4.1.1.

3. Evaluation of the application of arbuscular mycorrhizal fungi and magnetically treated water for the management of nematodes in protected culture conditions

Samples were processed in the provincial plant health laboratory, and the nematological analysis carried out on soil and roots showed densities of 40 Juveniles in their second stage (J2) per 100 cm^{-3} in soil and 130 J2 10 g^{-1} in roots. Once the perineal patterns were studied, the presence of the nematode *Meloidogyne incognita* was determined. Although there is the possibility of finding variability in morphometric parameters within the same species, which may be linked to environmental factors that directly influence the development of nematode populations, this way of identifying species is recognized by researchers [32].

3.1 Tomato cultivation *(Solanum lycopersicum)*

The results revealed that the use of AMF with pre-sowing inoculation is a practice with positive results; as the levels of pest infestation were reduced, the performance of the crop is even better when the AMF were combined (specifically *G. cubense* and *R. irregularis*) with MTW. *G. cubense* + MTW (0.1–0.12 T) provides the highest values of the means, although it does not statistically surpass *G. cubense* + MTW (0.05–0.07 T) (**Figure 1a–c**). This is because in addition to the effects exerted individually by both practices, it is added that, together, they show greater potential for crop development and a more effective response against nematode attacks.

Inoculation with AMF of plants that are subsequently infected by *Meloidogyne* allows nutrient uptake, plant growth, production of bioactive compounds and fruit production to increase. These benefits can extend over several cycles. In addition, it promotes complex physiological changes that can decrease the attraction of nematodes to the root. These physiological changes include the activation of defense mechanisms (elicitation), including increased activity of defense enzymes, increased production of nematicidal compounds, increased root lignification and alteration in cell wall composition, which can reduce the number of nematodes that penetrate and infect the roots [33].

The three AMF strains presented fungal functioning in relation to the control without inoculation and the treatments without inoculation + MTW. The trend is shown toward higher values of percentage of root colonization for *Glomus cubense* and *Rhizophagus irregularis* in combination with MTW, respectively, highlighting *Glomus cubense* + MTW (0.1–0.12 T). This may be due to the fact that, in the presence of MTW, the growth of AMF is stimulated, and at the same time, the plant's defense mechanisms are favored.

In the coffee plant (*Coffea arabica*) crop, AMF inoculation increases the root system and can reduce susceptibility and damage caused by nematodes [17]. The existence of

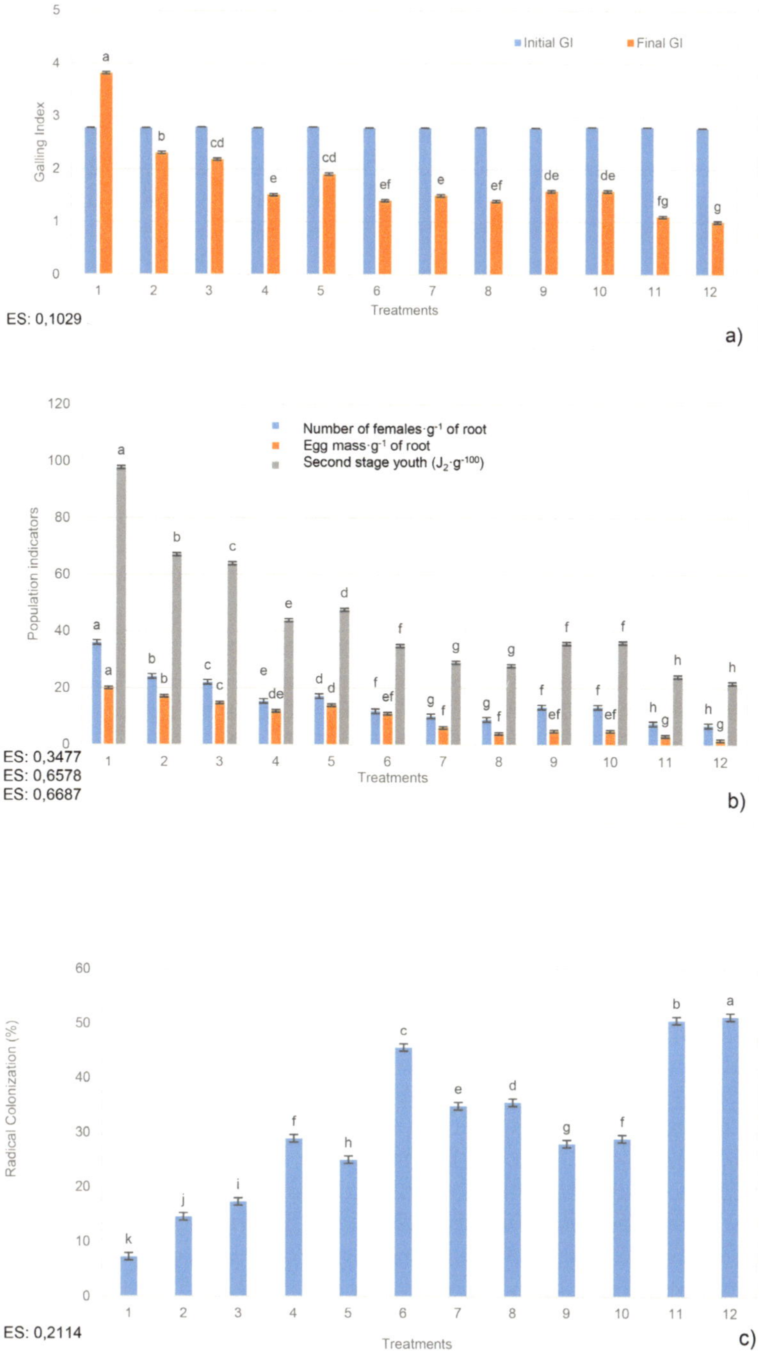

Figure 1.
Root galling index (a). Meloidogyne incognita *egg mass, number of females and juveniles J2 (b). Percentage of radical colonization of AMF (c) for tomato cultivation. 1: control without AMF inoculation; 2: culture without AMF + MTW inoculation (0.05–0.07 T); 3: culture without inoculation of AMF + MTW (0.1–0.12 T); 4:* Rhizophagus irregularis*; 5:* Funneliformis mosseae*; 6:* Glomus cubense*; 7:* Rhizophagus irregularis *+ MTW (0.05–0.07 T); 8:* Rhizophagus irregularis *+ MTW (0.1–0.12 T); 9:* Funneliformis mosseae *+ MTW (0.05–0.07 T); 10:* Funneliformis mosseae *+ MTW (0.1–0.12 T); 11:* Glomus cubense *+ MTW (0.05–0.07 T); 12: Glomus cubense + MTW (0.1–0.12 T).*

mechanisms such as greater absorption of nutrients, alteration of root morphology, competition for space and nutrients and induction of systemic resistance of the plant can contribute to improving the response of the plant to pest attack [34].

This result is determined by the pH in water (5.8–7.3) in which this process was developed since it was influenced by the neutralization of the bicarbonates contained in the irrigation water, which is more suitable for the normal development of the strains. The values could be given by the ability of efficient AMF strains to establish a molecular dialog with the macrosymbiont in close relationship with the edaphic environment of the soil and stimulate higher percentages of root occupancy. It is necessary to highlight the importance of the edaphic environment and pH on the effectiveness of AMF strains [35].

Mycorrhizae allow plants to absorb more phosphorus, nitrogen and water, improving their resistance to extreme environmental conditions. It also allows you to hinder the attack of pathogens that cause root diseases, protect the environment and completely avoid the use of agrochemicals. For its part, biocontrol using AMF arises from the need to look for alternatives that ensure protection for agriculture but at the same time do not have consequences on the environment. This has driven the search and development of new options for chemical agents [36].

It can be seen that considering the effects of AMF on plants attacked by nematodes, in most cases, a decrease in the severity of the infestation is observed, possibly due to the fact that plant-parasitic nematodes are antagonists, obligate biotrophs, like AMF. Likewise, it was proven that there is an antagonistic relationship caused by arbuscular mycorrhizal fungi toward pathogens and that the reduction of damage due to their attacks is not based solely on a greater number of roots [37, 38].

Numerous mechanisms are manifested when AMF promote biocontrol. They can be grouped into two: those that include a direct effect of the fungus on the pathogen such as competition for nutrients, space and infection/colonization sites and those that include indirect effects on the pathogen such as improvement in host nutrient uptake, changes in the architecture of the roots, changes in the interaction of rhizosphere microorganisms and activation of plant defense mechanisms [39].

The different mechanisms cannot be considered completely independent of each other, that is, the resulting biocontrol comes from a combination of several of them. Mechanisms include increased plant tolerance, direct competition for nutrients and space, induced systemic resistance and rhizosphere interactions [40].

Plants have defense systems against various stresses through the production of hormones, of small molecular weight, to activate their response/attack arsenal, and adapt to the new adverse condition. Salicylic acid (SA), jasmonic acid (JA) and ethylene (ET) are hormones which modulate the activation of defense genes for the immediate response against biotic stress (bacteria, fungi, insects, etc.) In general, against the attack of a biotrophic living pathogen (that feeds on living cells), plants defend themselves producing SA and alerting systemically to distal sites such as leaves, flowers and fruits (SAR), and this can be induced by AMF [41].

Plants are attacked by a multitude of pathogens and pests, some of which cause epidemics that threaten food security [42]. After infection by a pathogen, the colonization of roots with beneficial microorganisms such as AMF allows many plants to establish a physiological situation called "activated" or "primed" state. This allows them to respond more quickly and/or effectively when they are re-exposed to biotic or abiotic stress, a characteristic that is frequently associated with greater resistance to diseases.

There are also studies [43] that show that MTW provides greater tolerance to crop plants against pathogen attack. A decrease in the nematode root-knot index is also reported due to the influence of MTW, which improves the fitness of the plant that serves as host, as the plant has good vigor due to greater availability of nutrients [24]. Furthermore, in another investigation [22], they managed to increase yields by more than 10% with the use of magnetically treated water in tomato cultivation under protected cultivation house conditions.

Although the application of water treated with a magnetic field reduces the galling rate of *Meloidogyne*, it cannot be classified as a method of nematode control, as no mechanism has been found that can exert any control over the populations of the phytonematode, constituting a non-conventional alternative for phytosanitary protection against phytonematodes of the genus *Meloidogyne* due to the protection it confers on the crop [24].

Regarding the mechanisms that participate in this biological protection, they are not yet fully characterized. Other authors [44] argue that the effective "biological protection" against root pathogens, granted by AMF, is probably a consequence of several indirect mechanisms since they do not interact directly with pathogens through antagonism, antibiosis or parasitism. In the literature, [45, 46] propose several mechanisms: such as compensation of damage due to the better nutritional status of the host, anatomical and morphological changes of the root system that hinder the penetration of the pathogen, competition for colonization and infestation sites, competition for photosynthates, deposition in the rhizosphere of nematicidal and nematostatic metabolites, changes in soil microbial populations and activation of the plant defense response, induced resistance.

Various investigations have shown that the use of inoculation with AMF facilitates the absorption of water and nutrients, improves the physiological performance of crops attacked by nematodes, reduces stress and reduces the damage caused by this pest, which is why it is considered as a biological tool to be considered in a management plan [47, 48]. Furthermore, due to its characteristics, tomato tends to be frequently attacked by this pest [49, 50]. Plants interact with microorganisms, and these interactions have a notable impact on plant health. The oldest and most widespread mutualistic symbiosis between plants and microorganisms is that established with mycorrhizal fungi. Consequently, plants have evolved mechanisms to restrict pathogenic interactions while promoting mutualistic relationships.

The efficiency of these mechanisms depends on the adequate and timely recognition of the interacting fungi and the strict regulation of the immune responses triggered to control (promote or contain) fungal colonization. For example, nitric oxide (NO) acts as an intra- and intercellular signaling molecule. Involved in the regulation of many cellular functions in different species, NO produced after the recognition of pathogens by plants is part of the signaling cascades that trigger the expression of defense genes, the production of secondary metabolites and finally, hypersensitivity (HR) and systemic-acquired resistance (SAR) [51].

3.2 The cultivation of pepper *(Capsicum annuum)*

At the beginning of the investigation, the nematological analysis of the soil was carried out, which resulted in grade 1 of infestation; however, over the course of the experience, the control increased to grade 2.6, while treatments 2 and 3 without AMF inoculation presented grade 2, the other treatments (with AMF inoculation) showed galling rates below grade 2, the two treatments of *G. cubense* + MTW are the ones with the lowest rate with statistical differences to the other treatments which constitute a positive effect by providing the AMF and the magnetically treated water with greater tolerance to the crop to face the attack of nematodes (**Figure 2a–c**). The same behavior is observed in the population indicators of the nematode, as the treatments with *G. cubense* + MTW have the lowest average values, which demonstrate that the synergistic action of AMF and MTW causes a decrease in nematode populations.

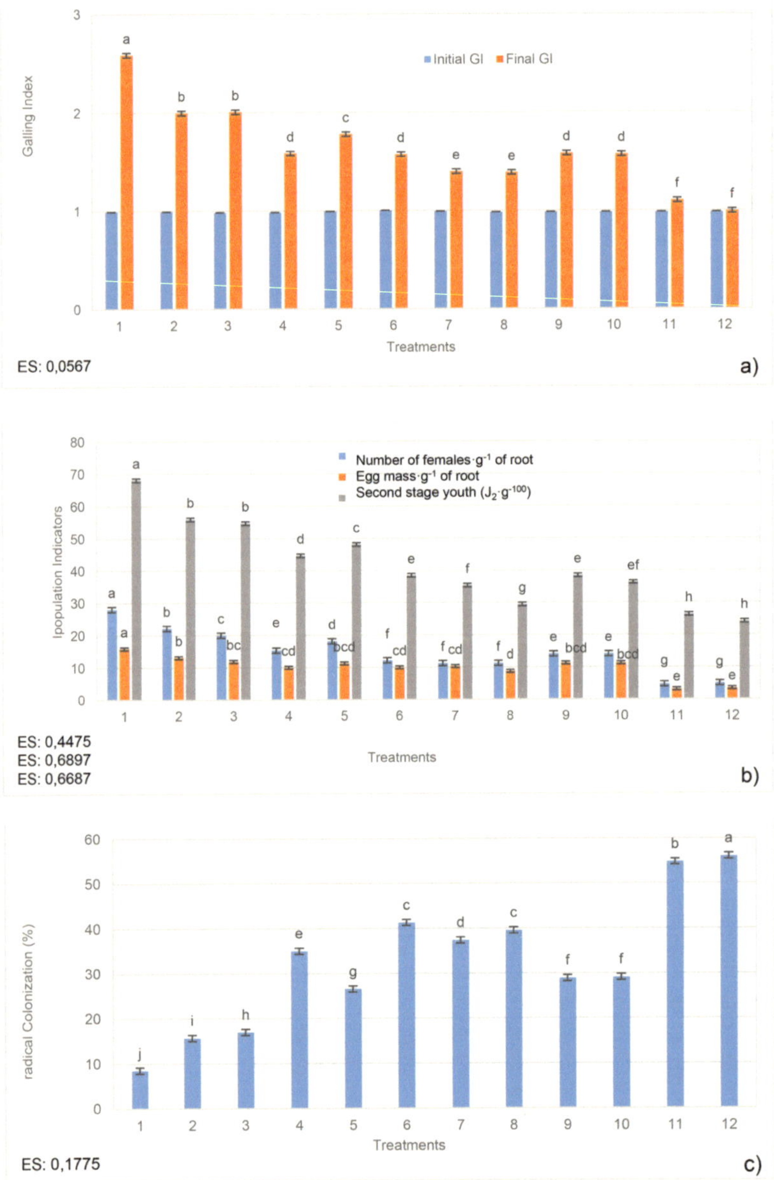

Figure 2.
Root galling index (a). Meloidogyne incognita *egg mass, number of females and juveniles J2 (b). Percentage of radical colonization of AMF (c) for the pepper crop. 1: control without AMF inoculation; 2: culture without AMF + MTW inoculation (0.05–0.07 T); 3: culture without inoculation of AMF + MTW (0.1–0.12 T); 4:* Rhizophagus irregularis*; 5:* Funneliformis mosseae*; 6:* Glomus cubense*; 7:* Rhizophagus irregularis *+ MTW (0.05–0.07 T); 8:* Rhizophagus irregularis *+ MTW (0.1–0.12 T); 9:* Funneliformis mosseae *+ MTW (0.05–0.07 T); 10:* Funneliformis mosseae *+ MTW (0.1–0.12 T); 11:* Glomus cubense *+ MTW (0.05–0.07 T); 12:* Glomus cubense *+ MTW (0.1–0.12 T).*

Authors such as in [52] propose that mycorrhizae, when establishing symbiosis with the roots of plants, emit their hyphae, which constitutes an elongation of the root system, providing it with a more favorable water and nutritional state compared to plants that are not mycorrhizal, which allows them to be able to face the impact of pathogens in a better situation. In his research [53], he points out that inoculated arbuscular mycorrhizal fungi managed to reduce the damage induced by the nematode, in *C. annuum*, with control effects superior to the chemical nematicide oxamil, improving the growth and agronomic vigor of the plants.

They also associate with plants and constitute a mutualistic relationship which is used in horticultural production, where they are implemented as a strategy to improve crop nutrition and reduce abiotic stress, and as biological control agents of root pathogens, they compete with nematodes for spaces in the root, modify the chemical composition of radical exudates that inhibits the penetration of J2 and activate defense mechanisms in plants [54, 55].

Regarding the percentage of radical colonization, the *Glomus cubense* + MTW treatment with the highest magnetic induction has the best result, statistically surpassing the other treatments, followed by the other combination of *Glomus cubense* and MTW, which is the control without inoculation of lower value than the average. Similar results were obtained [56], when evaluating the effectiveness of these strains in the cultivation of pepper in protected conditions, and for the same type of soil at pH levels of 7.2, the *Glomus cubense* strain stands out as the one that performed best.

It is suggested that the minimum percentage of AMF colonization should be greater than 40% to favor the symbiotic relationship with the plant and serve as a biological indicator of soil quality. The values could be given by the ability of efficient AMF strains to establish a molecular dialog with the macrosymbiont that is closely related to the type of soil and the pH level [57].

For its part, the authors of [58] demonstrated that treatments inoculated with *Glomus cubense* showed significantly higher percentages of mycorrhizal colonization, visual density and number of spores in the rhizosphere than those not inoculated for brown soils without carbonates. The above corroborates the effectiveness of this strain to achieve, at least under the conditions of this experiment, higher radical occupancy levels than native AMF. All these are added to the biostimulant effect of magnetically treated water that enhances the development of mycorrhization.

In a research carried out in pepper with another strain of AMF [59], they managed to reduce the population of nematodes, and with this, the reduction of damage to the roots, the reduction of the reproduction of the nematode and, in turn, the AMF favored the growth of the plants.

AMF have frequently been considered as a method to help the host plant attenuate damage caused by pathogens and predators [60]. In a study carried out by these authors, they evaluated the effects of a commercial AMF inoculum against *Meloidogyne incognita* in pepper. Under controlled conditions, the results were that the association of mycorrhizae decreased the development of *M. incognita* and improved tolerance to nematode infestation. These researchers suggest rapid mycorrhization of plants is essential to achieve protective effects against biotic stress.

The root-knot nematode *Meloidogyne incognita* causes galls on the roots of pepper resulting in yield losses. Although they recognize that the control of this pest in pepper with chemical nematicides is effective, there are environmental and health concerns that constitute serious drawbacks and limit their possible use [61]. They used four species of AMF in the cultivation of pepper in greenhouse conditions. They suggest using arbuscular mycorrhizal fungi to control this nematode as it may represent a solution to inhibit infestation by nematodes, improving the growth and fruit yield of this crop. Based on the results obtained, these AMF species could be used as biocontrol agents for *M. incognita*.

AMF are capable of improving plant growth by increasing the absorption of nutrients in exchange for photosynthetic carbon from their hosts, achieving successful biocontrol of nematodes as they reduce their population and reduce the number of galls, plants respond favorably in all parameters of growth and development, as well as showing an increase in yield [62].

It is generally recognized that arbuscular mycorrhizal fungi promote plant growth. Furthermore, they induce a defense response by plants against soil-borne pathogens such as plant-parasitic nematodes [63].

With mycorrhization, constant increases in plant weight are achieved, and it is recommended that root colonization by AMF should be established before nematode attack to ensure that prepared plants trigger effective immune action response capable of limiting the damage caused by infection [64]. Therefore, the optimal doses of the formulations, the age of the plant, the time between AMF inoculation and exposure to nematodes, soil type, growing conditions, etc., should be investigated and standardized to make of AMF treatment a successful and widespread component of integrated pest management in conventional and organic agriculture.

3.3 Cultivation of cucumber *(Cucumis sativus)*

When analyzing **Figure 3a–c**, which shows the *Meloidogyne incognita* galling index in each treatment in the cucumber crop and the percentage of root colonization by AMF, it can be seen that the treatments with AMF inoculation present the best behavior in the presence of the nematode *M. incognita* and manage to reduce galling to 1.5 in the case of the combination *G. cubense* + MTW, which statistically surpasses the control without inoculation, although they do not present significant differences with the other treatments. In the case of the percentage of root colonization, the behavior of the treatments with AMF inoculation statistically surpassed the treatments that do not present inoculation; however, the treatments with the *G. cubense* + MTW strain were the ones with the best results, although there were no differences among the inductions under study.

The use of AMF as an alternative for the control of root pathogens in horticultural crops is an area of study little explored in several countries. Among the main factors that are considered at the time of evaluation are the effect of AMF on nematodes to reduce their reproductive capacity, such as the estimate of reduction of eggs and females by the nematode and the severity of the damage it induces in the roots, where the number of galls and their arrangement on the root are considered, as well as their ability to promote crop growth considering this parasitic load [65].

AMF can reduce nematode development. Sustainable agriculture is currently promoted throughout the world, which guarantees human food security without negatively impacting the environment. AMF, naturally present in the soil and acting as biostimulators and bioprotectors, can be very beneficial for sustainable agriculture, maintaining plant production and reducing pathogens without harming the environment. Given the importance of sustainable crop management and the lack of studies specifically addressing the interactions of AMF and *Meloidogyne*, it is important to conduct research [33].

The biocontrol characteristics of arbuscular mycorrhizal fungi (AMF) against root pathogens are known, but information on the mode of biocontrol action and biocontrol efficiency of AMF species is limited. In general, it is considered that the biocontrol characteristics of AMF in terms of tolerance induction depend on the AMF species. These differential traits of AMF should be considered when developing biocontrol strategies against cucumber root pathogens [66].

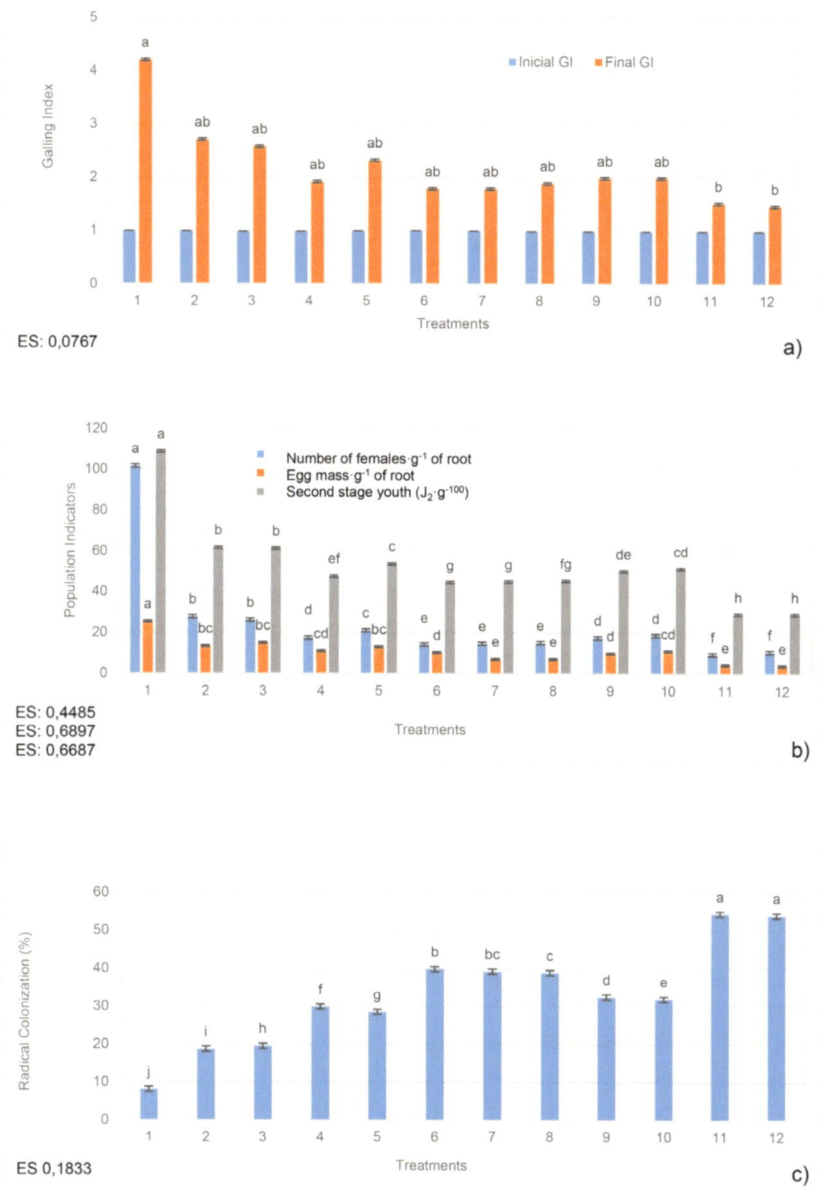

Figure 3.
Root galling index (a). Meloidogyne incognita *egg mass, number of females and juveniles J2 (b). Percentage of radical colonization of AMF (c) for cucumber cultivation. 1: control without AMF inoculation; 2: culture without AMF + MTW inoculation (0.05–0.07 T); 3: culture without inoculation of AMF + MTW (0.1–0.12 T); 4:* Rhizophagus irregularis*; 5:* Funneliformis mosseae*; 6:* Glomus cubense*; 7:* Rhizophagus irregularis *+ MTW (0.05–0.07 T); 8:* Rhizophagus irregularis *+ MTW (0.1–0.12 T); 9:* Funneliformis mosseae *+ MTW (0.05–0.07 T); 10:* Funneliformis mosseae *+ MTW (0.1–0.12 T); 11:* Glomus cubense *+ MTW (0.05–0.07 T); 12:* Glomus cubense *+ MTW (0.1–0.12 T).*

Treatments inoculated with *Glomus cubense* showed significantly higher percentages of mycorrhizal colonization in the rhizosphere than those not inoculated for brown soils without carbonates [67]. The above corroborates the effectiveness of this strain to achieve, at least under the conditions of this experiment, higher radical occupancy levels than native AMF. Other authors [68] state that another group of potential fungi in the biocontrol of nematodes is that of arbuscular mycorrhizal fungi (AMF), which function as obligate symbionts of plant roots. The plant provides photosynthetic carbon for symbionts, while helping roots absorb more nutrients and stimulating both root growth and leaf structure.

Furthermore, AMF often compete for nutrition and space with these soil pathogens and induce systemic plant resistance. Also, the authors of [69–71] state that plants can still be immunized against nematode attacks through beneficial microorganisms of the rhizosphere, such as arbuscular mycorrhizal fungi that can induce systemic responses of acquired resistance against nematodes.

3.4 The cultivation of chard *(Beta vulgaris var. cicla)*

When analyzing **Figure 4a–c**, it can be seen that, in the control (where mycorrhizae was not applied), there was an increase in the nematode galling index with an average of 3.50, if it is considered that the initial galling index was 3. The two treatments consisting of the application of MTW (with the two inductions under study) also showed effects by nematodes; however, in the rest of the treatments, the means were 0, which statistically exceeds the control and the treatments without AMF + MTW inoculation.

This seems to be motivated by the protective effect exerted by mycorrhizae in their symbiosis with plant roots. It is also proposed that the action of AMF minimizes the physiological damage caused by nematodes [72]. The increase in the percentage of root colonization could be caused by the actions exerted by AMF in the increase and absorption of nutrients available for plants. This increase could be the result of competition between AMF and nematodes for root space. This would stimulate the growth of intraradical mycelium, favor its development and increase colonization levels.

With the use of arbuscular mycorrhizal fungi (AMF), it is inferred that the participation of these associated with agricultural crops can influence the dynamics of mineral elements such as copper, zinc, iron and manganese, reflected in the concentration in their plant tissue through the homeostasis of heavy metals and their transcriptional activity, which is why it biofortifies vegetables, especially leafy ones such as chard, and this adds to the already known benefits that these microorganisms provide [73].

Antagonistic microorganisms such as AMF have mechanisms that regulate nematode population densities, so culture-independent and culture-dependent approaches have been adopted and used in several studies to analyze the diversity of bacteria or fungi associated with nematode genera plant parasites [74].

Related to this [75], it is stated that soil biota performs a series of functions that are essential for the integrity and productivity of agricultural systems, which is why it constitutes a fundamental part of terrestrial biodiversity. The composition of this biota can be manipulated, almost always temporarily, to maintain and increase the productivity of a soil.

AMF in combination with MTW act on the plant and enhance the induced systemic resistance. During their life, plants interact with numerous pests, which have different modes of attack and life forms. The primary immune response evolved toward the recognition of organisms that interact with the plant and the translation of such recognition into defense responses specifically directed against the invading organism. This type of resistance often acts systemically and is effective against a wide spectrum of pests [76].

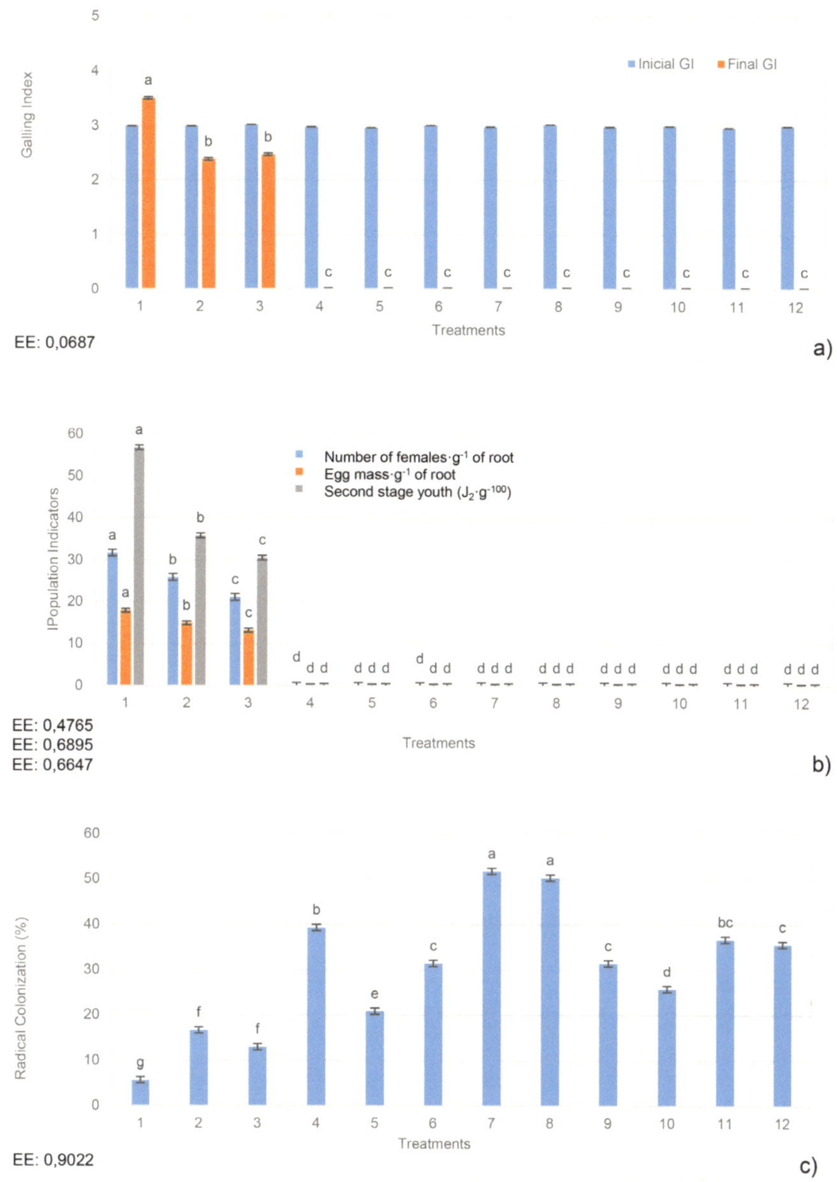

Figure 4.
Root galling index (a). Meloidogyne incognita *egg mass, number of females and juveniles J2 (b). Percentage of radical colonization of AMF (c) for the Swiss chard crop. 1: control without AMF inoculation; 2: culture without AMF + MTW inoculation (0.05–0.07 T); 3: culture without inoculation of AMF + MTW (0.1–0.12 T); 4:* Rhizophagus irregularis*; 5:* Funneliformis mosseae*; 6:* Glomus cubense*; 7:* Rhizophagus irregularis *+ MTW (0.05–0.07 T); 8:* Rhizophagus irregularis *+ MTW (0.1–0.12 T); 9:* Funneliformis mosseae *+ MTW (0.05–0.07 T); 10:* Funneliformis mosseae *+ MTW (0.1–0.12 T); 11:* Glomus cubense *+ MTW (0.05–0.07 T); 12:* Glomus cubense *+ MTW (0.1–0.12 T).*

The use of beneficial microorganisms is a viable alternative for production since they constitute an economically attractive and ecologically acceptable medium. They reduce external inputs, improve the quantity and quality of internal resources, as well as guarantee greater efficiency in the use of mineral fertilizers [77].

4. Conclusions

AMF considerably reduces the formation of galls and the reproductive capacity of the nematode in tomato, pepper, cucumber and chard crops.

Irrigation with MTW enhances the positive effects of AMF in the management of *M. incognita*, which demonstrates that its combined use can be a beneficial alternative for the management of nematodes in crops grown under protected cultivation conditions.

Author details

Daniel Rafael Vuelta Lorenzo[1]*, Siannah María Más Diego[2], Gerardo Montero Limonta[1] and Miriela Rizo Mustelier[1]

1 Departamento de Agronomía, Facultad de Ingeniería Química y Agronomía, University of Oriente, Santiago de Cuba, Cuba

2 Centro Nacional de Electromagnetismo Aplicado, University of Oriente, Santiago de Cuba, Cuba

*Address all correspondence to: dvuelta@uo.edu.cu

References

[1] Huerta K, Martínez A, Colón A. La revolución verde. Revista Iberoamericana de Bioeconomía y Cambio Climático. 2018;**4**:8, 1040-1062. DOI: 10.5377/ribcc.v4i8.6717

[2] Raza A, Razzaq A, Mehmood SS, Zou X, Zhang X, Lv Y, et al. Impact of climate change on crops adaptation and strategies to tackle its outcome: A review. Plants. 2019;**8**(2):1-29. Article 34. DOI: 10.3390/plants8020034

[3] Delgado-Zegarra J, Alvarez-Risco A, Yáñez JA. Uso indiscriminado de pesticidas y ausencia de control sanitario para el mercado interno en Perú. Revista Panamericana de Salud Pública. 2018;**42**:e3. DOI: 10.26633/RPSP.2018.3

[4] Peña-Prades M, Olivares-Reyes N, Rodríguez-Regal M, Peña-Rivera L, Cobas- Elías A, Cervera-Duverger G, et al. Nematodos fitoparásitos asociados al cultivo de la caña de azúcar (*Saccharum officinarum* L.) en la provincia Guantánamo, Cuba. Cultivos Tropicales. 2018;**39**(1):7-14

[5] Rodríguez-Carnero OJ, Rodríguez M, Puchades Y, La O-García JC, Lora-Reyes N, Lodo-Vega Z, et al. Inventario de la nematofauna asociada al cultivo de la caña de azúcar (*Saccharum sp*) en Santiago de Cuba. Ciencia en su PC. 2020;**1**(3):92-107

[6] Quesada-Mola Y, Fernández-Gonzálves E, Casanueva-Medina K, Ponce-Grijuela E, Márquez- Gutiérrez ME. Actividad biológica de nuevas cepas cubanas de Tríchoderma spp. efectivas en el control de *Meloidogyne incognita* (Kofoid & White) Chitwood. Revista Cubana de Ciencias Biológicas. 2019;7(1):NA

[7] Miranda Cabrera I, Hernández-Ochandía D, Hernández del Amo Y, Martínez Coca B, Rodríguez Hernández MG. Modelación de la interacción *Meloidogyne incognita* (Kofoid y White) Chitwood- Trichoderma asperellum Samuels, Lieckfeldt & Nirenberg en garbanzo (Cicer arietinum L.). Revista de Protección Vegetal. 2016;**31**(3):194-200

[8] Patil JA, Yadav S. Root-knot nematodes a major peril to protected cultivation system in India: Current status and its management. In: Bellé C, Kaspary TE, editors. Nematodes—Recent Advances, Management and New Perspectives. IntechOpen; 2022. DOI: 10.5772/intechopen.94719

[9] Castillo N, Díaz D, García O, Marrero O. Influencia de Tecnologías alternativas de fertilización en el rendimiento agrícola de los cultivos Tomate (*Solanum lycopersicon* L), Lechuga (*Lactuca sativa* L) y Pimiento (*Capsicum annuum*, L.). Innovación Tecnológica. 2020;**26**(4):1-15

[10] Vuelta-Lorenzo DR, Rizo-Mustelier M, Aroche-Alarcón JA. Empleo de alternativas para el manejo de nemátodos en el cultivo del tomate (*Solanum lycopersicum*) en la finca Santo Tomás. Ciencia en su PC. 2019;**1**(1):1-15

[11] Altier N, Abreo E. Una sola salud: Consideraciones en el Año Internacional de la Salud Vegetal. Agrociencia (Uruguay). 2020;**24**(spe):1-14

[12] Lopez, Nicora H, Soilan Duarte LC, Grabowski Ocampos CJ, Enciso Maldonado GA, Caballero Mairesse GG. Manual de Nematología agrícola: bases y procedimientos. Editorial Atlas. 2021:1-90. DOI: 10.53997/DFXA5914

[13] Vallejos-Torres G, Arévalo L, Iliquin I, Solis R. Respuesta en Campo

de Clones de Café a la Inoculación con Consorcios de Hongos Micorrízicos Arbusculares en la Región Amazonas, Peru. Información Tecnológica. 2019;**30**(6):73-84. DOI: 10.4067/S0718-07642019000600073

[14] Urgiles-Gómez N, Guachanamá-Sánchez J, Granda-Mora I, Robles-Carrión Á, Encalada- Cordova M, Loján-Armijos P, et al. Caracterización morfológica de hongos micorrízicos arbusculares (HMA) asociados al café en sistemas agroforestales de la provincia de Loja, Ecuador. Bosques Latitud Cero. 2020;**10**(2):137-145

[15] Ojeda L, Rodríguez Y. Efecto de la inoculación con Hongos Micorrízicos Arbusculares y humus de lombriz en el establecimiento de un banco forrajero de Pennisetum purpureum VC. Taiwan morado. Revista Científica Agro-Ecosistemas. 2018;**6**(2):86-91

[16] Saparrat M, Bernardo V, Ruscitti M, Elíades L, Balatti P. Hongos rizosféricos y el movimiento del fósforo en el suelo. In: Saparrat M, Ruscitti M, Arango M, editors. Micorrizas arbusculares: biología y aplicaciones en el sector agro-forestal. 1ra ed. Libro digital, PDF - (Libros de cátedra) La Plata: EDULP; 2020

[17] Trejo-Aguilar D. Efecto de la micorriza arbuscular en plantas de café (*Coffea arabica* L.) Infectadas por el nematodo de la corchosis de la raíz. Agro Productividad. 2018;**11**(4):98-107

[18] Simó-González JE, Ruiz-Martínez LA, Rivera-Espinosa R. Inoculación de hongos micorrizógenos arbusculares (HMA) y relaciones suelo pardo-abonos orgánicos en la aclimatización de vitroplantas de banano. Cultivos Tropicales. 2017;**38**(3):02-111

[19] Faggioli V, Symanczik S. Servicios eco-sistémicos provistos por hongos formadores de micorrizas y efecto de las prácticas de manejo en cultivos de base agroecológica. In: Ullé J, Diaz BM, editors. El suelo como reactor de los procesos de regulación funcional de los agroecosistemas. Vol. 3. Argentina, Capitulo: INTA Ediciones; 2018. pp. 87-106

[20] Anaya M, Barbará E, Padrón J, Borrego SF, Valdés O, Molina A. Influencia del campo magnético sobre el crecimiento de microorganismos patógenos ambientales aislados en el Archivo Nacional de la República de Cuba. Biomédica. 2015;**35**(3):325-336

[21] Boix YF, Dubois AF, Alemán EI, Victório CP, Arruda R d C d O, Cuypers A. Static Magnetic Treatment of Irrigation Water on Differents Plants Cultures Improving Development. Vol. 35 (Santos CC, Ed.). Ponta Grossa, Paraná, Brasil: Atena Editora; 2019. pp. 76-84

[22] Zamora-Oduardo D, Rodríguez-FernándezP,Ferrer-DuboisAE,Fung-BoixY, Isaac-Aleman E, Asanza-Kindelán G. Producción de tomate (*Solanum lycopersicum* L.) bajo riego con agua magnetizada en casa de cultivo protegido. Ciencia en su PC. 2020;**1**(1):60-74

[23] Elías-VigaudY,Rodríguez-FernándezP, Fung-Boix Y, Isaac-Aleman E, Ferrer-Dubois A, Asanza-Kindelán G. Producción de pepino (*Cucumis sativus* L.) en casa de cultivo semiprotegido bajo riego con agua magnetizada. Ciencia en su PC. 2020;**1**:75-86

[24] Quiala RA, Isaac E, Simón FA, Regueiferos I, Montero G. Efecto del agua tratada con campo magnético estático sobre *Meloidogyne* spp. en *Cucumis sativus* en condiciones de cultivo protegido. Centro Agrícola. 2011;**38**(4):83-87

[25] Murad S, Jabbar A, Gad S. Efficiency of using magnetized water in improving *Meloidogyne incognita* control by three

concentration of *Aloe vera* extract on cucumber plant. Plant Archives. 2019;**19**:721-727

[26] Hassan H. Effect of magnetized water with some nano-preparations on tomato plants infection with the root knot nematode *Meloidogyne javanica*. Egyptian-Arab Journal of Applied Sciences and Technology. 2022;**2**(2):11-14. DOI: 10.21608/eajast.2022.128365.1009

[27] Hassan H, Tantawy M, Younes A, Sayed M. The role of magnetized water in root- knot nematode integrated management programs associated with grapevines in Minia governorate. Journal of Modern Research. 2023;**5**(2):50-52. DOI: 10.21608/jmr.2023.195449.1103

[28] Bolaños, Benavides MM, Jaramillo Noreña JE, Ropero Barbosa L, Peña Holguin AC, Montes ML, León RI, et al. Innovaciones para la horticultura en ambientes protegidos en zonas cálidas: opción de intensificación sostenible de la horticultura familiar en el contexto del cambio climático en América Latina y el Caribe (ALC). FONTAGRO (Fondo Regional de Tecnología Agropecuaria). 2022;**5**:1-40

[29] Fernández F, Vanega L, Noval B, Rivera R. Producto inoculante micorrizógeno. Instituto Nacional de Ciencias Agrícolas. Oficina Nacional de Propiedad Industrial. Cuba. No. 22641. 2000

[30] Jaramillo NJ, Rodríguez PV, Guzmán AM, Zapata M, Rengifo MT. Manual Técnico: Buenas Prácticas Agrícolas en la Producción de tomate bajo condiciones protegidas. 2007. 331 p

[31] Casanova AS, Hernández JC. Manual para la producción protegida de Hortalizas. 3ra ed. La Habana (VE): Editorial Liliana Djmitrova; 2023

[32] Artavia-Carmona R, Peraza-Padilla W. Identificación morfológica, morfométrica y molecular de *Meloidogyne exigua* (Göeldi 1887) en café (*Coffea arabica*). Agronomía Mesoamericana. 2020;**31**(3):531-545

[33] da Silva Campos MA. Bioprotection by arbuscular mycorrhizal fungi in plants infected with *Meloidogyne* nematodes: A sustainable alternative. Crop Protection. 2020;**135**:105203. DOI: 10.1016/j.cropro.2020.105203

[34] Forghani F, Hajihassani A. Recent advances in the development of environmentally benign treatments to control root-knot nematodes. Frontiers in Plant Science. 2020;**11**:1125. DOI: 10.3389/fpls.2020.01125

[35] Rivera R, Ruiz L, Martin G, Pérez E, Nápoles MC, García M, et al. Manejo conjunto e impacto de biofertilizantes micorrízicos y otros bioproductos en la producción agrícola de diferentes cultivos. Informe Primer Semestre Junio 2015. Cuba: Instituto Nacional Ciencias Agrícolas; 2015

[36] García-Nieto DA, Marín-Cevada V, Reyes-Montes T. Protegiendo al jitomate: *Biocontrol al día. Alianzas y Tendencias*—BUAP. 2020;**5**(17):1-14

[37] Contreras JR, Mercado D. Micorrizas arbusculares: antagonistas naturales de los patógenos del suelo. Revista Agroexcelencia. Capaciagro. México. 2019;**24**(1):22-24

[38] Ahamad L, Bhat AH, Kumar H, Rana A, Hasan MN, Ahmed I, et al. From soil to plant: Strengthening carrot defenses against *Meloidogyne incognita* with vermicompost and arbuscular mycorrhizal fungi biofertilizers. Frontiers in Microbiology. 2023;**14**:1206217

[39] Dar MH, Reshi ZA. Vesicular Arbuscular Mycorrhizal (VAM) fungi as a major biocontrol agent in modern sustainable agriculture system. Russian Agricultural Sciences. 2017;**43**(2):138-143. DOI: 10.3103/S1068367417020057

[40] Schouteden N, De Waele D, Panis B, Vos CM. Arbuscular mycorrhizal fungi for the biocontrol of plant-parasitic nematodes: A review of the mechanisms involved. Microbiology. 2015;**6**:1280. DOI: 10.3389/fmicb.2015.01280

[41] León-Reyes A, Barriga N. Memorias del 4to Simposio en Fitopatología, Control Biológico e Interacciones Planta-Patógeno. Archivos Académicos USFQ. 2019;**23**:107-107

[42] Maya, Álvarez MÁ. Caracterización y control de plagas en áreas edificadas y ajardinadas. SEAG0110. España: IC Editorial; 2023

[43] Elaoud A, Ben Salah N, Jalel R, Turki N. Evaluation of the effect of the magnetic apparatus on the water, the plant and the state of the soil. International Journal of Engineering and Technology. 2019;**9**(4):529-531

[44] Azcón-Aguilar C, Jaizme-Vega MC, Calvet C. The contribution of arbuscular mycorrhizal fungi to the control of soil-borne plant pathogens. In: Gianinazzi S, Schüepp H, Barea JM, Haselwander K, editors. Mycorrhizal Technology in Agriculture. Switzerland: Brikhäuser Verlag; 2002. pp. 187-197

[45] Azcón-Aguilar C, Barea JM. Arbuscular mycorrhiza and biological control of soil-borne plant pathogens— An overview of the mechanisms involved. Mycorrhiza. 1996;**6**:457-464

[46] Harrier LA, Watson CA. The potential role of arbuscular mycorrhizal (AM) fungi in the bioprotection of plants against soil-borne pathogens in organic and/or other sustainable farming systems. Pest Management Science. 2004;**60**:149-157

[47] Bernardo V, Garita S, Arango C, Ripodas J, Saparrat M, Ruscitti M. Arbuscular mycorrhizal fungi against the false root-knot nematode activity in *Capsicum annuum*: Physiological responses in plants. Biocontrol Science and Technology. 2020;**31**(2):119-131. DOI: 10.1080/09583157.2020.1833304

[48] Garita SA, Bernardo VF, Gonzalez M, Ripodas JI, Arango MC, Ruscitti M. The false root-knot nematode: Modification of the root anatomy and alteration of the physiological performance in tomato plants. Rhizosphere. 2021;**20**:100424

[49] Aquino-Bolaños T, Matadamas-Ortíz PT, Lopez-Vasquez CF, Ines-Vasquez S. Management of the nematode of the nodule of *Meloidogyne incognita* in tomato (*Solanum lycopersicum* L.) with extracts in a biospace condition. African Journal of Agricultural Research. 2019;**14**:180-184. DOI: 10.5897/AJAR2018.13602

[50] Inés-Vásquez S, Aquino-Bolaños T. Biocontrol y Tolerancia de *Meloidogyne incognita* en Tomate. Southwestern Entomologist. 2020;**45**(4):957-963. DOI: 10.3958/059.045.0413

[51] Terrón-Camero LC, Molina-Moya E, Peláez-Vico MÁ, Pescador Azofra L, Martínez-Medina A, Pozo Jiménez MJ, Sandalio L, Romero-Puertas MC. Nitric Oxide Role in Plant-Fungi Interactions. España: Universidad Internacional de Andalucía; 2021

[52] Morales L, Rodríguez J, Jerez E, Estrada W. Efecto de dos bioestimulantes y hongos micorrízicos en plantas de tomate sembradas a altas temperaturas. Cultivos Tropicales. 2018;**39**(3):41-48

[53] Herrera-Parra E, Cristóbal-Alejo J, Zavala-León MJ, Basto-Pool CI. Hongos micorrícicos arbusculares y Trichoderma en *Capsicum annuum* disminuyen el daño inducido por *Meloidogyne incognita*. Temas Agrarios. 2023;**28**(1):37-45. DOI: 10.21897/rta.v28i1.3158

[54] Diagne N, Ngom M, Brahima DP, Fall D, Hocher V, Svistoonoff S. Roles of arbuscular mycorrhizal fungi on plant growth and performance: Importance in biotic and abiotic stressed regulation. Diversity. 2020;**2**(10):370. DOI: 10.3390/d12100370

[55] Weng W, Yan J, Zhou M, Yao X, Gao A, Ma C, et al. Roles of arbuscular mycorrhizal fungi as a biocontrol agent in the control of plant diseases. Microorganisms. 2022;**10**(7):1266. DOI: 10.3390/microorganisms10071266

[56] Toledo B, Montero G, Bazán A. Efecto de la inoculación con hongos micorrízicos arbusculares (HMA), en el rendimiento del Pimiento (*Capsicum annum* L.) bajo condiciones protegidas. Agrisost. 2020;**26**(1):1-12

[57] Pérez Y, Álvarez JD, Mendoza J, Pat JM, Gómez R, Cuevas L. Diversidad de hongos micorrízicos arbusculares en maíz con cultivo de cobertura y biofertilizantes en Chiapas, Mexico. Botánica. 2012;**69**(1):46-56

[58] Michels-Mighty J, Rodríguez-Fernández P, Montero-Limonta G. Producción de pimiento (*Capsicum annum* L.) en casa de cultivo protegido con fertirriego e inoculación con *Glomus cubense*. Ciencia en su PC. 2020;**1**:18-30

[59] Herrera-Parra E, Ramos-Zapata J, Basto-Pool C, Cristóbal-Alejo J. Sweet papper (*Capsicum annuum*) response to the inoculation of native arbuscular mycorrhizal fungi and the parasitism of root-knot *Meloidogyne incognita*. Revista Bio Ciencias. 2021;**8**:e982. DOI: 10.15741/revbio.08.e982

[60] Rodríguez-Heredia M, Djian-Caporalino C, Ponchet M, Lapeyre L, Canaguier R, Fazari A, et al. Protective effects of mycorrhizal association in tomato and pepper against *Meloidogyne incognita* infection, and mycorrhizal networks for early mycorrhization of low mycotrophic plants. Phytopathologia Mediterranea. 2020;**59**(2):377-384

[61] Udo IA, Akpan JF, Bello OS, Otie VO. Arbuscular mycorrhizal fungus species differed in bio-control potential on pepper genotypes infected with *Meloidogyne incognita*. International Journal of Vegetable Science. 2023;**29**(3):261-274

[62] Razek G, Abdelaziz S. Effect of arbuscular mycorrhizal fungi and some plant growth promoting rhizobacteria in controlling root-knot nematode (*Meloidogyne incognita*) on tomato under greenhouse conditions. Egyptian Journal of Desert Research. 2019;**69**(3):131-150

[63] Molinari S, Akbarimotlagh M, Leonetti P. Tomato root colonization by exogenously inoculated arbuscular mycorrhizal fungi induces resistance against root-knot nematodes in a dose-dependent manner. International Journal of Molecular Sciences. 2022;**23**(16):8920

[64] Udo IA, Uko AE, Obok EE, Ubi JO, Umoetok SB. Management of *Meloidogyne* incognita and salinity on sweet pepper (*Capsicum annuum* L.) with different arbuscular mycorrhizal fungus species. Journal of Applied Biology and Biotechnology. 2022;**10**(4):66-72

[65] Cristóbal-Alejo J, Ramos-Zapata J, Basto-Pool C, Herrera-Parra E. Hongos micorrícicos arbusculares como control biológico del nematodo agallador (*Meloidogyne* spp.) en hortalizas de Yucatán. Bioagrociencias.

2021;**14**(1):11-17. DOI: 10.56369/BAC.3692

[66] Ravnskov S, Cabral C, Larsen J. Mycorrhiza induced tolerance in *Cucumis sativus* against root rot caused by Pythium ultimum depends on fungal species in the arbuscular mycorrhizal symbiosis. Biological Control. 2020;**141**:104133

[67] Reyes, Pérez JJ, Rivero Herrada M, Andagoya Fajardo CJ, Beltrán Morales FA, Hernández Montiel LG, García Liscano AE, et al. Emergencia y características agronómicas del *Cucumis sativus* a la aplicación de quitosano, *Glomus cubense* y ácidos húmicos. Biotecnia. 2021;**23**(3):38-44. DOI: 10.18633/biotecnia.v23i3.1427

[68] Abd-Elgawad MMM. Optimizing safe approaches to manage plant-parasitic nematodes. Plants. 2021;**10**:1911. DOI: 10.3390/plants10091911

[69] El-Nagdi WMA, Youssef MAM, Abd-El-Khair H, Abd-Elgawad MMM. Effect of certain organic amendments and *Trichoderma* species on the root-knot nematode, *Meloidogyne incognita* infecting pea (*Pisum sativum* L.) plants. Egyptian Journal of Biological Pest Control. 2019;**29**:75

[70] Zipfel C, Oldoryd GED. Plant signalling in symbiosis and immunity. Nature. 2017;**543**:328-336

[71] Gao X, Guo H, Zhang Q. Arbuscular mycorrhizal fungi (AMF) enhanced the growth, yield, fiber quality and phosphorus regulation in upland cotton (*Gossypium hirsutum* L.). Scientific Reports. 2020;**10**:2084

[72] Gómez, Tovar L. Manual de Sistemas Hortícolas Diversificados. México: Universidad Autónoma de Chapingo; 2021

[73] Gío-Trujillo JA, Alvarado-López CJ, Pacheco-López NA, Cristóbal-Alejo J, Reyes-Ramírez A. Perspectivas futuras de la biofortificación de alimentos: la asociación con microorganismos del suelo. Ra Ximhai. 2022;**18**(4):175-199

[74] Dongmei Z, Feng H, Schuelke T, Santiago A, Zhang Q, Zhang J, et al. Rhizosphere microbiomes from root knot nematode non-infested plants suppress nematode infection. Microbial Ecology. 2019;**78**:470-481. DOI: 10.1007/s00248-019-01319-5

[75] Habte M. The roles of arbuscular mycorrhizas in plant and soil health. In: Biological Approaches to Sustainable Soil Systems. EUA: Boca Ratón; 2006

[76] Peteira Delgado-Oramas B. La resistencia inducida como alternativa para el manejo de plagas en las plantas de cultivo. Revista de Protección Vegetal. 2020;**35**(1):e07

[77] León González Y, Martínez Viera R, Dibut Álvarez B, Hernández Martínez JM, Hernández GB. Factibilidad económica de la aplicación de inoculantes microbianos en el cultivo del tabaco negro. Cultivos Tropicales. 2016;**37**(1):28-33